Ketogenic Diet:

The Best Ketogenic Recipes to Lose Weight

Jessica Moore

Table of Contents

Introduction 7

Keto Breakfast 9

Recipe #1: Southwest Omelets.................................10

Recipe #2: Keto Pancakes 12

Recipe #3: Keto English Breakfast 14

Recipe #4: Ricotta Oatmeal 16

Recipe #5: Bulletproof Coffee 18

Recipe #6: Coffee Mug Muffin.................................20

Recipe #7: Feta/Pesto Omelet 22

Recipe #8: Keto Porridge 24

Recipe #9: Avocado Boats..26

Recipe #10: Keto Waffles 28

Keto Lunch 30

Recipe #11: Caprese Salad....................................... 31

Recipe #12: Keto Bacon-Wrapped Stuffed Jalapeños 33

Recipe #13: Keto Tuna Salad 35

Recipe #14: Thai Tuna Salad 36

Recipe #15: A Proper Crust......................................38

Recipe #16: Taco Pie..40

Recipe #17: Spinach Feta Quiche 42

Recipe #18: Cheesy Broccoli Soup 44

Recipe #19: Burger Bowl...46

Recipe #20: New York Frittata.................................48

Keto Dinner..50

Recipe #21: Keto Pizza (Option 1) 51

Recipe #22: Keto Pizza (Option 2)...........................53

Recipe #23: Mushroom Bun Burger 55

Recipe #24: Keto Red Curry 57

Recipe #25: Keto Mac and Cheese Cauliflower Casserole 59

Recipe #26: Eggplant Lasagna 61

Recipe #27: Chicken Pesto Casserole.................................63

Recipe #28: Keto Chicken Curry 65

Recipe #29: Baked Salmon 67

Recipe #30: Keto Asian Skillet 69

Keto Snacks 71

Recipe #31: Chocolate Peanut Butter Fat Bombs 72

Recipe #32: Cheesy Broccoli.................................73

Recipe #33: Kale Chips 75

Recipe #34: Keto Onion Dip 77

Recipe #35: Keto Burger Bombs 79

Recipe #36: Mediterranean "Guacamole" 81

Recipe #37: Neapolitan Fat Bombs.................................83

Recipe #38: Keto Deviled Eggs.................................85

Recipe #39: Bacon-Smoked Gouda Stuffed Mushrooms .87

Recipe #40: Keto Nacho Chips.................................89

Keto Desserts 91

Recipe #41: Low Carb Cheesecake 92

Recipe #42: Coconut Cocoa Cookies.................................93

Recipe #43: Delicious Peanut Butter Balls 95

Recipe #44: Keto Chocomocha Mousse.................................97

Recipe #45: Keto Pound Cake 98

Recipe #46: Lemon Poppyseed Soufflé.................................100

Recipe #47: No-Bake Coconut Almond Bars.................................102

Recipe #48: Hot Chocolate Mug Cake 103

Recipe #49: Peanut Butter Cookies................................105

Recipe #50: Pumpkin Pie Pudding 106

Conclusion...108

© Copyright 2017 by Jessica Moore - All rights reserved.

The following eBook is reproduced below with the goal of providing information that is as accurate and reliable as possible. Regardless, purchasing this eBook can be seen as consent to the fact that both the publisher and the author of this book are in no way experts on the topics discussed within and that any recommendations or suggestions that are made herein are for entertainment purposes only. Professionals should be consulted as needed prior to undertaking any of the action endorsed herein.

This declaration is deemed fair and valid by both the American Bar Association and the Committee of Publishers Association and is legally binding throughout the United States.

Furthermore, the transmission, duplication or reproduction of any of the following work including specific information will be considered an illegal act irrespective of if it is done electronically or in print. This extends to creating a secondary or tertiary copy of the work or a recorded copy and is only allowed with an express written consent from the Publisher. All additional rights reserved.

The information in the following pages is broadly considered to be a truthful and accurate account of facts, and as such any inattention, use or misuse of the information in question by the reader will render any resulting actions solely under their purview. There are no scenarios in which the publisher or the original author of this work can be in any fashion deemed liable for any hardship or damages that may befall them after undertaking information described herein.

Additionally, the information in the following pages is

intended only for informational purposes and should thus be thought of as universal. As befitting its nature, it is presented without assurance regarding its prolonged validity or interim quality. Trademarks that are mentioned are done without written consent and can in no way be considered an endorsement from the trademark holder.

Introduction

Congratulations on purchasing *Ketogenic Diet: The Best Ketogenic Recipes to Lose Weight* and thank you for doing so.

There are tons of healthy cookbooks available in the market that offer weight loss recipes. Each book guarantees good health and slim physique. Most of these diet books require you to cut away your favorite foods and force you to eat those that you do not like. Also, the programs are rather short-lived and do not offer long term benefits.

Many people today commit themselves to spending their wealth and time to trying out different diet plans. They spend hundreds to thousands of dollars for various diet programs just to achieve their physical goal. Some people succeed in their goal, but most are barely seeing result.

The problem with diet cookbooks is that they will force you to change your eating habit and will make you eat foods that you have never been fond of. And frankly, breaking or changing your eating habit is very difficult. That's one of the reasons why dieters fail in achieving their goal. But the truth is, you do not have to give up your favorite food just to lose weight and achieve a slim, healthy body.

Ketogenic Diet is a new diet that's becoming very popular. Not just because it has helped many to lose weight, but also because it treats several physical illnesses. Another good thing about this diet is that you do not have to give up your favorite dishes.

This book is going to go through a lot of tantalizing, yummy ketogenic recipes. Not good at cooking? Fret not. The recipes contain easy-to-follow step by step guides that will make you feel like an expert keto chef. Sometimes, keto can get pretty monotonous - the goal of this book is to break that monotony and have you enjoying your food right away!

There are plenty of books on this subject on the market, thanks again for choosing this one! Every effort was made to ensure it is full of as much useful information as possible. Please enjoy!

Keto Breakfast

Breakfast is, without a doubt, the most important meal of the day! In this chapter, we're going to be covering a lot of the different things that you can prepare for a delicious ketogenic breakfast! Some of these are going to be a bit more complex while others are a bit simpler. Go at your own pace in deciding what works for you!

Recipe #1: Southwest Omelets

This is a really simple recipe. You can prepare everything in one pan, which makes it super simple to clean up, as well. This is called the Southwest omelet because it has a pleasant kick to it. This is really easy to make. Here's how you go about making this delicious and tasty breakfast!

What You Need:

- 3 eggs
- shredded Fiesta blend cheese
- 6 to 8 strips raw bacon
- white onion, chopped
- jalapeños, fresh, sliced, NO SEEDS
- salsa
- sour cream

How to Prepare:

1. Start by cooking raw bacon to your desired doneness. When the bacon is ready, set it to the side and then pour the excess drippings into a container. This is a habit you want to get into as a keto dieter, because the drippings are not only delicious but are a natural product of the animals you're using and a useful fat,

as well. When cooled enough, dice bacon into small strips.

2. Coat pan with bacon drippings and heat on stove to medium or medium-high. In a separate bowl, scramble your eggs and add salt, pepper, cream or any other desired agents. Once eggs are scrambled, and the pan is sufficiently hot, dump the eggs into the pan.

3. The goal here is for the eggs to cook all the way through and also make a bit of a tortilla shape. While you wait for the egg to start to firm all the way through, throw in your jalapeños, bacon strips, and white onion so it all cooks into the egg.

4. Once the egg has firmed up, spread a liberal amount of cheese on top and throw some jalapeños on top of it. Then, layer the jalapeños with even more cheese in order to add a locking layer. Close the tortilla egg into a bit of a taco or omelet shape, then flip in order to cook on both sides. Continue flipping as necessary until interior white is fully cooked.

5. Remove from heat and enjoy! Garnish with salsa, sour cream, and/or hot sauce as desired.

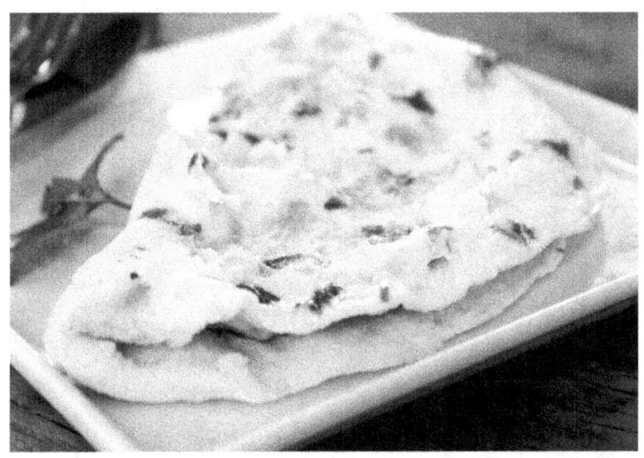

Recipe #2: Keto Pancakes

This is a simple but tasty recipe that will fill a vacancy in your low-carb life that leaves you without delicious flaky pancake goodness. This tastes a little bit like French toast, or potentially fried cheesecake! Either way, it's really good. Pair it with sugar-free maple syrup for a tasty combination that will get your mornings off to a great start. Here's how you make it.

What You Need:
- 2 ounces of high-quality cream cheese
- 2 eggs
- Artificial sweetener of your choice
- Cinnamon
- Vanilla extract

How to Prepare:

1. Blend all of your ingredients together in a fine pancake-like "batter" is ready. Much like real pancakes or crêpes, you don't have to cook very much at once for these things to be delicious, so a little goes a long way.
2. Get out a pan and put it on a burner over medium-high heat. Melt either butter or coconut oil in the pan to grease it.
3. Again, much like pancakes and crêpes, you don't have to go crazy with this; when the pan is appropriately hot, just dump a bit in there and spread it thin, then cook it on either side. Much like real pancakes, let these cook a little before you try to flip them. Trying to flip them too early could result in pancake catastrophe! (Or at least a few broken pieces.)
4. Serve with butter and sugar-free maple syrup. Enjoy!

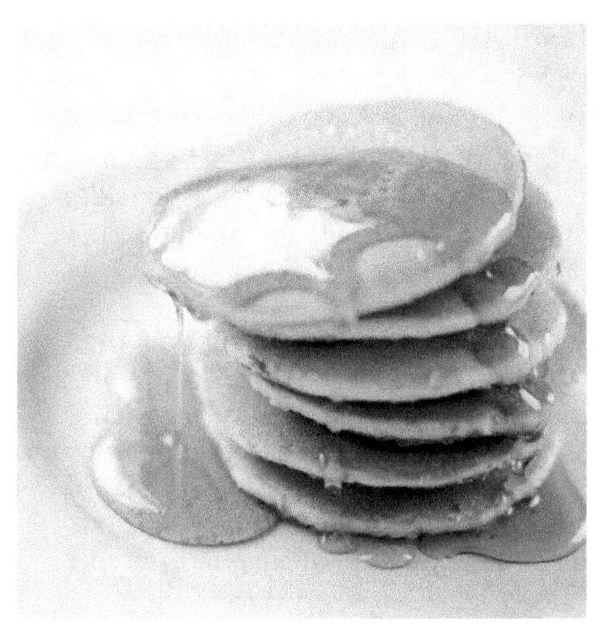

Recipe #3: Keto English Breakfast

Whether you call it the full English breakfast or simply a fry-up, this is a delicious meal that ports pretty well to keto and packs a lot of calories in it, too. You can serve it alongside English breakfast tea with half-and-half and Splenda for an authentic experience!

One of the joys of the fry-up is that all of the juices of the various foods cook together. Some of the things are a bit hard to find in America, so you will need to replace them with other things. The beans also are not acceptable. In other words, we'll largely be improvising here. However, all of the grease in the fry-up we'll be making serves you a delicious breakfast you'll be keen to have again and again.

What You Need:

- Mushrooms, chopped
- Tomato, sliced
- 3 sausage links
- 6 strips bacon
- 3 eggs
- black pudding, if you can find it

How to Prepare:

1) First, prepare your bacon strips - the fat will come in handy.
2) After, grill your mushrooms in the bacon fat. When the mushrooms are grilled, move on to the tomatoes.
3) When the tomatoes are grilled, throw your sausage links on. After the sausage links are finished, grilled your black pudding.
4) Use the residual fat and a tad bit of butter in order to fry your eggs sunny side up.

5) Serve everything on the plate individually. Combine
   while eating for maximum effect.

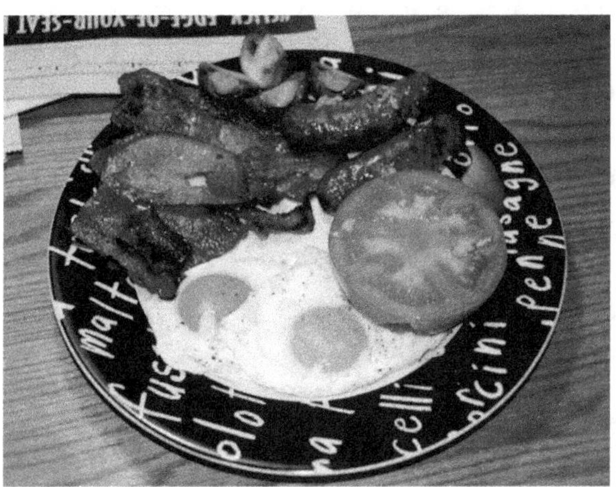

Recipe #4: Ricotta Oatmeal

This recipe is a delicious accent to your mornings. It gives you a pleasant oatmeal texture but doesn't require you to do anything particularly special. In fact, you can just microwave everything and have a delicious breakfast in less than a minute. Keto can be pretty demanding, so having an easy recipe like this is an absolute godsend! Do remember, though, that your ricotta cheese must be high-quality. Cheap or generic ricotta cheese often comes loaded with carbs from added sugars. Natural ricotta cheese can have as little as one carb per serving.

What You Need:

- ¾c ricotta, local if at all possible (lower carb than others)
- ⅓c salted organic butter
- cinnamon
- 4tbsp Splenda

How to Prepare:

1. Mix everything together in a microwavable bowl.
2. Stir once more before serving, then enjoy your delicious not-oatmeal oatmeal!

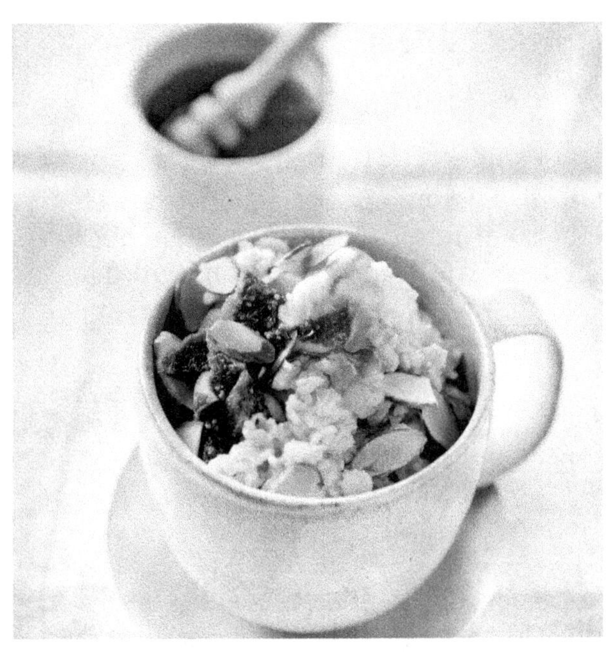

Recipe #5: Bulletproof Coffee

This is a really conventional ketogenic breakfast. If you don't know what Bulletproof coffee is, essentially, it's a combination of MCT oils and organic unsalted butter. This recipe doesn't exactly ask you to go that far, though. MCT oils are really just a concentrated form of coconut oil. This recipe is really simple and filling, and will also leave you with plenty of energy throughout your morning.

What You Need:
- Organic grass-fed unsalted butter
- High-quality coconut oil
- The best coffee you can find

Throw everything together in a blender. Since this is so simple, you really should try to get the best ingredients possible to maximize taste. Most people don't add anything to Bulletproof coffee, but if you need a quick and energizing breakfast and can't seem to get over the taste, you can add an artificial sweetener in order to make it more palatable.

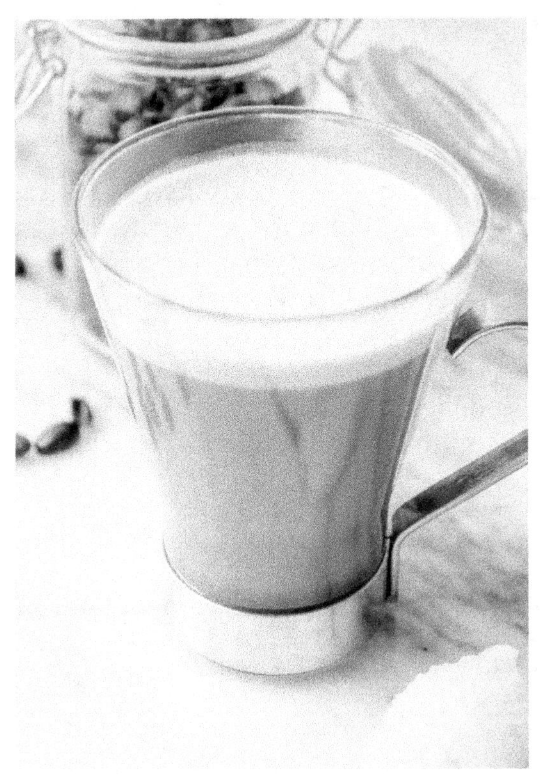

Recipe #6: Coffee Mug Muffin

This one is really simple! It doesn't have a whole lot of taste on its own, but the beauty is that it provides you a blank canvas to which you can add pretty much anything you want. Add a bunch of cinnamon or pumpkin spice and artificial sweetener, or maybe some blueberries and maple syrup. Potentially try making it savory and throwing cheese and meat within it.

One way or another, these delicious muffins will be a delicious and simple cornerstone of your keto breakfasts. Just give it a try!

What You Need:

- 2 eggs
- ½ cup flaxseed meal
- 2tsp of baking powder
- ¼ cup of milk
- 2tsp of sweetener
- 2tsp of vanilla
- 1tsp of cinnamon

How to Prepare:
- Combine everything in a large bowl.
- Pour into two mugs and microwave for 90 seconds each.
- You're done! Cool them and enjoy however you'd like.

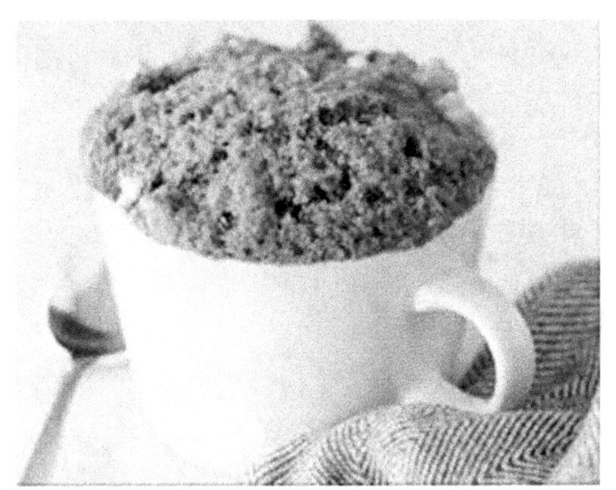

Recipe #7: Feta/Pesto Omelet

This one's really simple! It's yet another delicious omelet recipe. One thing you'll discover throughout this book is that I really, really love myself some feta. This recipe is the first manifestation of that deep love for this incredible cheese. This omelet is ridiculously easy to make.

What You Need:

- 3 eggs
- heavy cream (to fluff the eggs)
- butter
- 1tbsp of basil pesto
- 1oz feta

How to Prepare:

1. Use the butter in order to grease your pan - heat it in a medium pan over medium-high heat.
2. In a separate bowl, just like before, whisk your eggs, add your heavy cream, and add salt and pepper to your eggs. Not too much salt, though - feta has a lot by itself!
3. Throw your eggs in the greased pan. Let them cook mostly, just like before. Then spread your pesto all over one half of the egg. Top your pesto spread with your feta.
4. Fold the omelet into halves again and let the cheese melt.
5. There you go! All done. Garnish however you like and enjoy your delicious feta omelet.

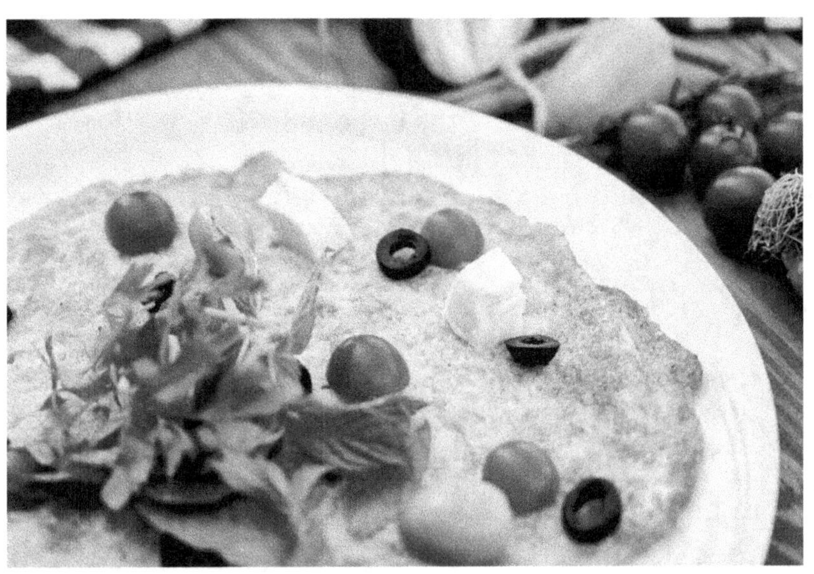

Recipe #8: Keto Porridge

This recipe is different from the last one in that it *acts* a lot more like oatmeal. It's not just a thick sweet cheese. It's actually a delicious choice for your morning that offers you the ability to add whatever you want.

What You Need:

- 2 cups of unsweetened almond milk
- 4tsp artificial sweetener
- ½ cup of flaxseed meal
- ½ cup of coconut flour
- 2tsp vanilla
- 2tsp cinnamon
- salt

How to Prepare:

1. Warm a pot over low heat and put your 2 cups of almond milk in it.
2. Add in all of your dry ingredients, then bring to a low boil.
3. Add in vanilla. Keep boiling until desired thickness, then remove from the flame.
4. Add what you like and enjoy it! This makes four servings.

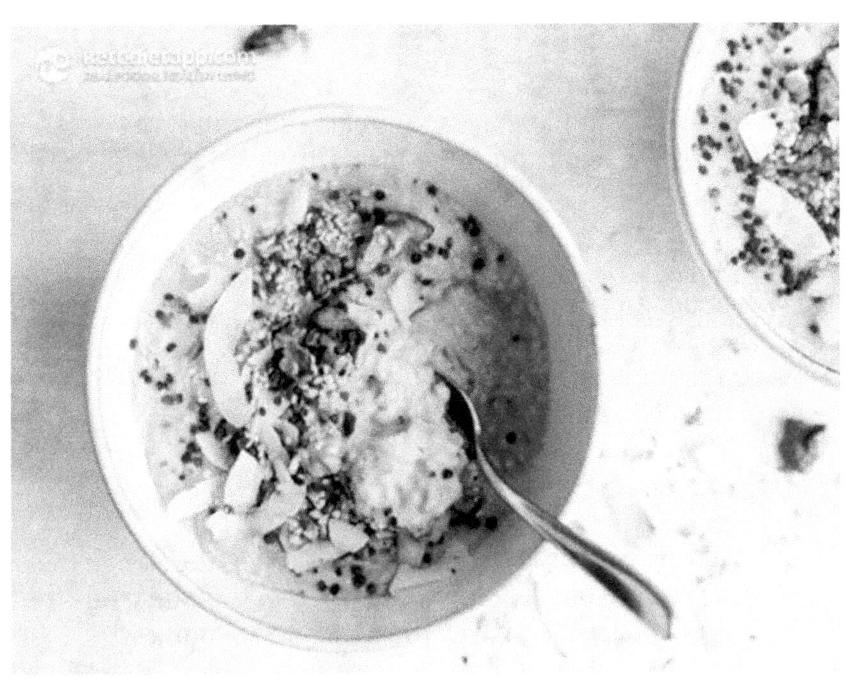

Recipe #9: Avocado Boats

These are super simple and tasty treats that will give you a super filling and healthful breakfast with very little effort on your end.

What You Need:
- 1 avocado per person
- 2 eggs per person
- Garlic salt
- Parmesan cheese (grated)

How to Prepare:

1. Start by warming your oven to 350 degrees.
2. Cut your avocados down the middle, then take out the pits. Take out a little of the avocado so that a whole egg can fit in each half.
3. Sprinkle your garlic salt on the avocado halves, as well as a bit of pepper. Go according to taste.
4. Crack an egg into each avocado half where you've carved out a place.
5. Sprinkle your parmesan over the egg, a healthy amount.
6. Throw in the oven and bake for 13 or 14 minutes.
7. Remove them from the oven and enjoy! This is a roughly 700 calorie breakfast, so it's more than enough energy to push you through the day.

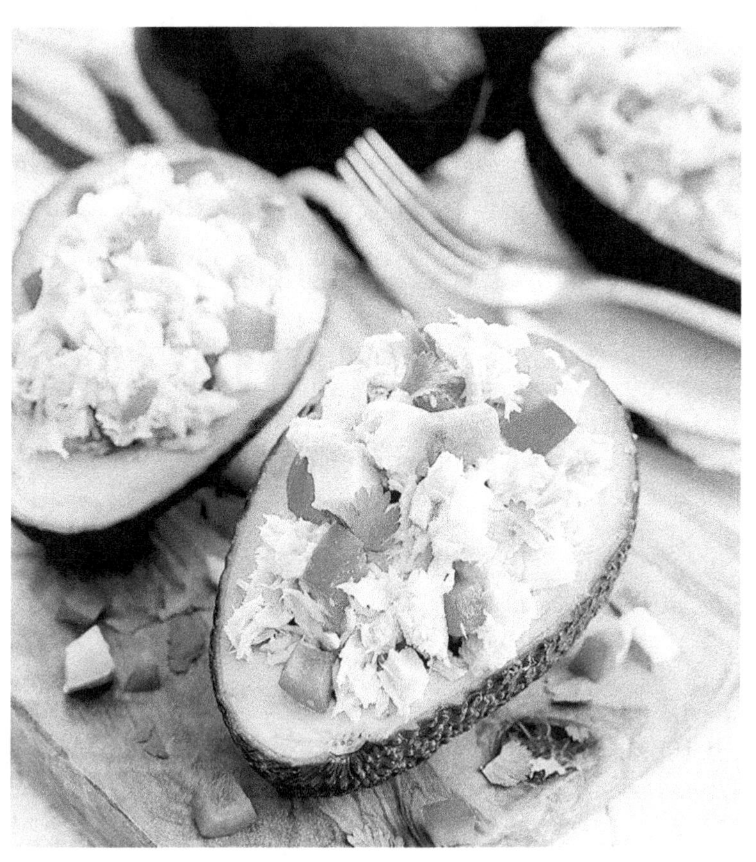

Recipe #10: Keto Waffles

These are super easy to make and allow you to get familiar
with a few materials that you'll start to be using a lot later
when you start making pie crusts and things of that nature.
Believe it or not, most things have a pretty handy "port" in
keto, and you won't have a whole lot of difficulty taking
things that you already like and then moving them over to
your ketogenic lifestyle. Much like normal waffles, you can
take these, pour the batter into the waffle maker, and then
top them with butter and syrup. They are, in effect, delicious
ketogenic waffles. Try them for yourself!

What You Need:

- 8 eggs
- 6tbsp of almond flour
- 2tbsp psyllium husk powder
- ½tsp vanilla
- 2tsp sweetener (Stevia and Splenda work well)
- 2tsp cinnamon
- 2tsp baking powder

How to Prepare:

1. Combine everything in a large bowl, then whisk
   together by hand or blend using an immersion
   blender. Blend until it starts to thicken.
2. Cook this on a waffle maker, just like you would a
   normal waffle. Start pouring it in and then just wait
   for it to be finished cooking. (Be careful not to open
   too early - just like normal waffles, they may not hold
   together very well in this case!)
3. Each waffle is finished when it's cooked like a normal

waffle would be. Top it with whatever you want. You can even use fresh cream and blueberries if you'd like! Then gobble them down. You won't be able to hold back!

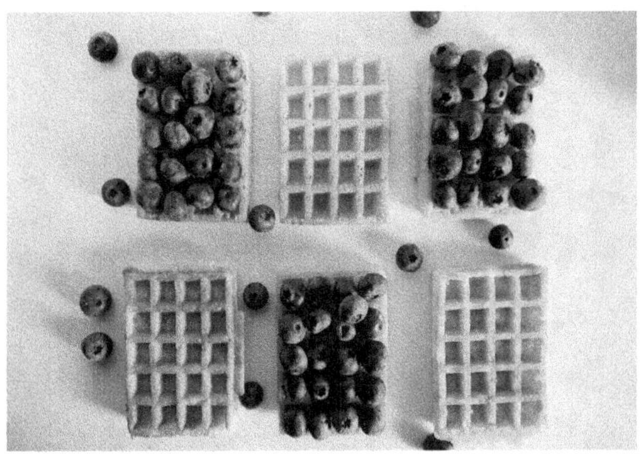

Keto Lunch

Recipe #11: Caprese Salad

This recipe is really simple. It's actually pretty much exactly
the one that you could get from street vendors in Italy, with
no substitutions. Tomatoes aren't high in carbs at all, and
you can get away with slicing and eating a tomato each day if
you so desire. Here's a fun fact - when this recipe was
created, the colors were specifically chosen to represent the
colors of the Italian flag. How cool is that!

What You Need:

-   High-quality mozzarella cheese (spring for organic
    and locally-produced if possible, as the quality will be
    much higher)
-   High-quality tomato (slicing tomatoes will do, but
    obviously, go for the best possible tomato that you
    can)
-   Basil leaves
-   Extra virgin olive oil

Slice your mozzarella cheese and tomato relatively thin and
start to arrange on a plate in sequence with the basil leaves,
so that the three can be easily paired. Top your dish with a
light salting and a healthy drizzle of olive oil.

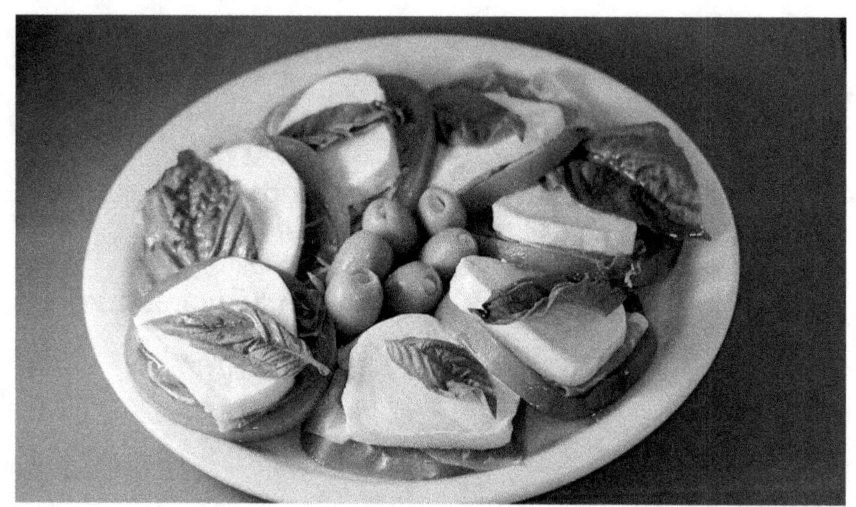

Recipe #12: Keto Bacon-Wrapped Stuffed Jalapeños

If you want a little kick in your lunch, then these bacon-wrapped stuffed jalapeños will be the perfect treat for you! They're extremely easy to make, and they're spicy enough to invigorate you when the lunchtime lull hits.

What You Need:

- 6 jalapeños, sliced in half lengthwise
- 6 slices of bacon sliced in half horizontally
- 8 ounces of cream cheese
- 1 packet of Ranch seasoning

How to Prepare:

1. Melt your cream cheese as much as you can using a microwave. After it's been melted, add your packet of Ranch seasoning to it.
2. Preheat your oven to 325 degrees.
3. Making sure that you've removed any remaining seeds or stems within the halved jalapeños, start to spread the cream cheese and ranch mixture inside them. This serves as a delicious filling.
4. Take one of your bacon halves and wrap it around each stuffed pepper. This will simultaneously hold in the cream cheese filling and, well, give you the delicious taste of bacon.
5. Place your twelve jalapeños on a foil-lined baking sheet and put in the oven. Cook until bacon is finished, roughly 20 minutes.
6. Remove your stuffed peppers from the oven and then chow down!

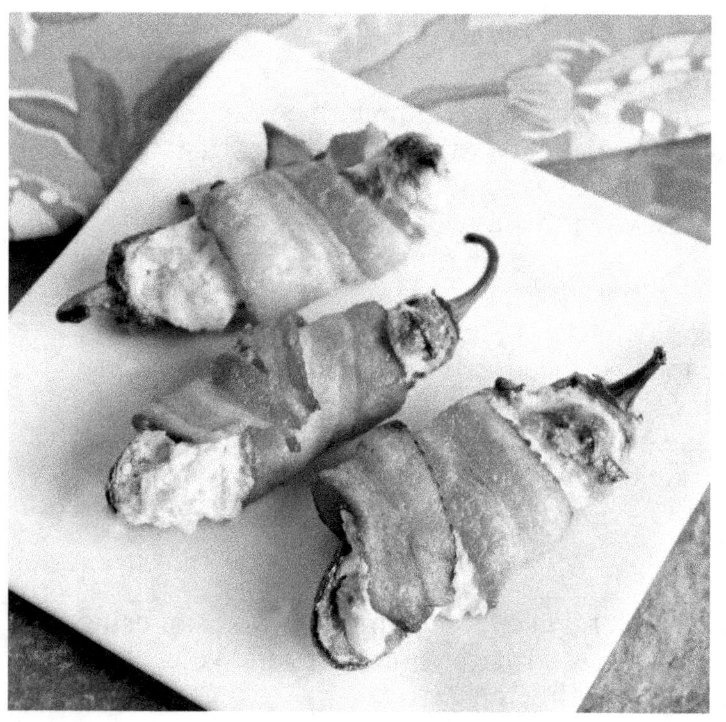

Recipe #13: Keto Tuna Salad

This is a pretty simple recipe to make, but it tastes very good. You can also make keto bread with it and toast that and enjoy your keto tuna salad on a bread mimic. One way or another, you're going to have a tasty and keto friendly tuna salad.

What You Need:

- 4 strips of bacon, cooked
- 2 cans worth of tuna
- 2 boiled eggs
- 1.5tbsp of Dijon Mustard
- 2tbsp Mayo
- 2tsp onion powder
- 2tbsp sour cream
- ½ tsp dill

1. Chop your cooked bacon up finely. Do the same for the egg.
2. Open your cans of tuna and then make sure there's no liquid.
3. Put your tuna in a mixing bowl. Add your bacon, eggs, and onion powder. Mix by hand to incorporate all. It should be a rough mixture.
4. Add your mayonnaise, sour cream, Dijon, and dill and use these to bind everything else.
5. When finished, sit back and enjoy your creation! Tasty.

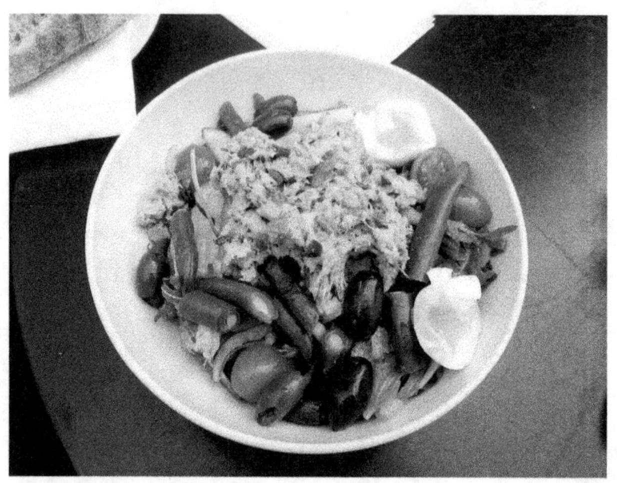

Recipe #14: Thai Tuna Salad

This one builds on the last recipe but gives it a little bit of a different edge to it! Give it a try!

What You Need:

- 6 cans worth of tuna
- 2 bell peppers
- 1 red onion
- 2 cucumbers
- ½ cup sesame oil
- 2 limes worth juice

How to Prepare:

1. Dice all of your vegetables! This is important.
2. Drain your tuna and then put them in a bowl. Break them apart into tinier tunas.
3. Add all of your vegetables, then your sesame oil, then the lime juice. Mix everything as well as you can.

4. Add salt/pepper as you wish.
5. That's all! You can garnish as you want, perhaps with mint or Thai basil if you can find any. Enjoy it! It makes approximately 8 servings.

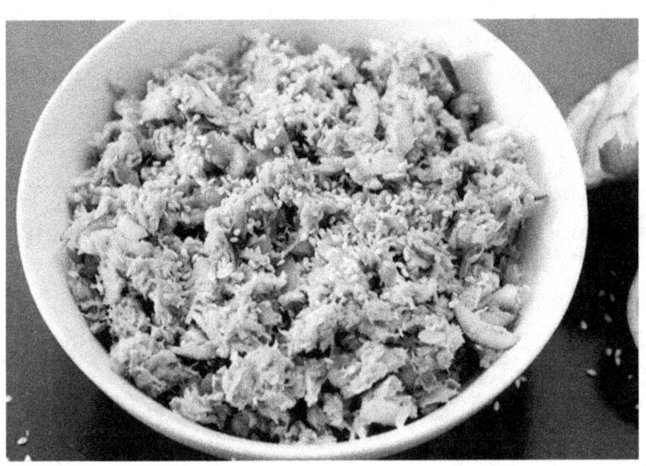

Recipe #15: A Proper Crust

This really shouldn't be its own recipe... however, it's extremely versatile, and you can use it in many different recipes, including the recipes which follow. In order to save space and keep from telling you how to make the same crust over and over, I'm just going to tell you how to make this one right now. There are a lot of ways to make crusts on keto. This is partially because there is no real *crust*, there are just things which are *crust-like*, and these are generally pretty simple to make. They're also a lot more difficult to get wrong than non-keto crusts, which is nice, and you don't have to wait for yeast to activate or anything.

In other words, if you learn this crust once, you can use it over and over again. That's exciting! So here it is.

What You Need:

- 1 cup of almond flour
- 2tbsp ground psyllium husk powder
- 6tbsp sesame seeds
- ¾ cup of coconut flour
- ¼ cup of flaxseed meal
- 2 eggs

How to Prepare:

1. Start by preheating your oven to 350 degrees. Combine all pie crust ingredients in food processor. Dough will be very firm.
2. Spread dough into greased pan. Perhaps use parchment paper in order to make it easier to loosen later. You can also use a springform pan. This makes a lot of dough, so you may not need it all.
3. Some recipes will require you to brown the dough first

while others won't. If that's the case, bake it for 15 minutes. Otherwise, just add your normal ingredients to it.

4. That's it! Now let's put this to use for some quality lunches.

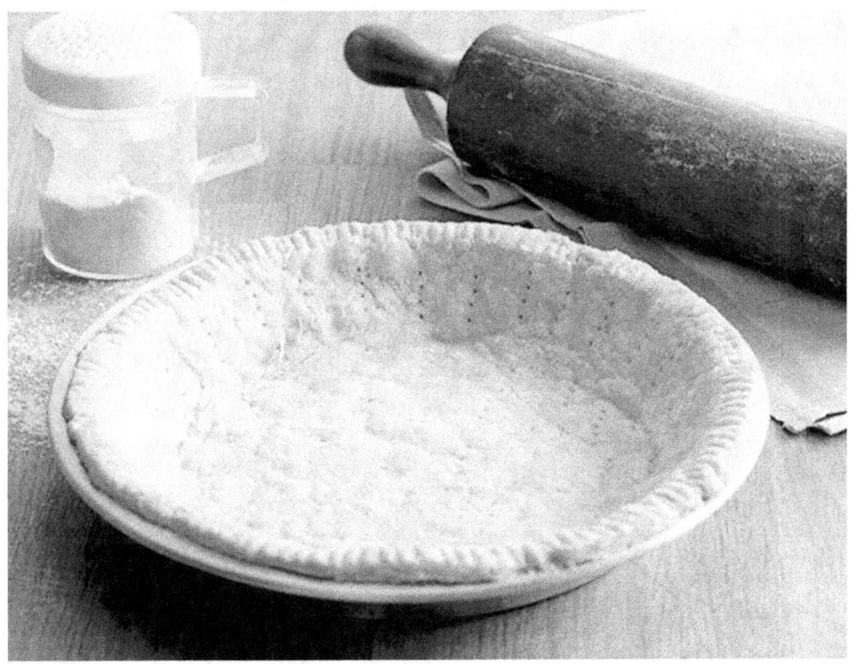

Recipe #16: Taco Pie

This is a really easy recipe. It uses the pie dough that we just developed as a base. Everything else is built around that. You can make this ahead of time and take it to work in Tupperware, then warm it up. It will last three or four days in the fridge. You don't need to brown it ahead of time, just make it and coat the bottom of the dish.

What You Need:

- Pie shell (already made)
- Ground beef, about a pound will do
- A packet of taco seasoning
- 5 eggs
- ½ yellow onion, chopped
- 1 clove garlic, minced
- ¾ cup cream
- 1 cup Fiesta blend cheese

How to Prepare:

1. Preheat your oven to 350 degrees.
2. Warm a skillet and brown your ground beef. While that's cooking, take the time to prepare your onion and garlic.
3. When the ground beef has been browned, combine all of the ingredients in a large bowl, then transfer it to the top of your pie crust. Top with a healthy amount of extra Fiesta blend cheese.
4. Bake for 25 to 30 minutes until the cheese is sufficiently browned.

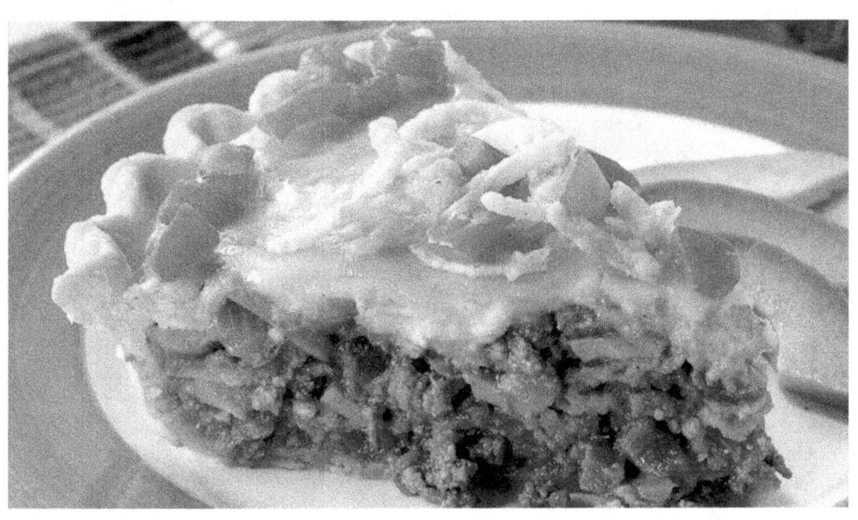

Recipe #17: Spinach Feta Quiche

I hope that by now you're starting to see the utility of the pie crust! Here's another that takes spinach and feta - one of my favorite combinations, remember! - and makes it into a delicious quiche that you can take to work over and over and never get tired of!

What You Need:

- Pie shell (already made)
- 2lb spinach
- 7oz feta cheese
- 8 eggs
- ½ yellow onion, chopped
- ¼ cup cream
- 8oz mushrooms, chopped

How to Prepare:

1. Preheat your oven to 350 degrees once again.
2. Mix everything thoroughly. Beat your eggs, season with salt and pepper as you like, and then just combine everything. Then dump it all into your pie shell.
3. Bake for 25 to 30 minutes. Be careful not to overcook!

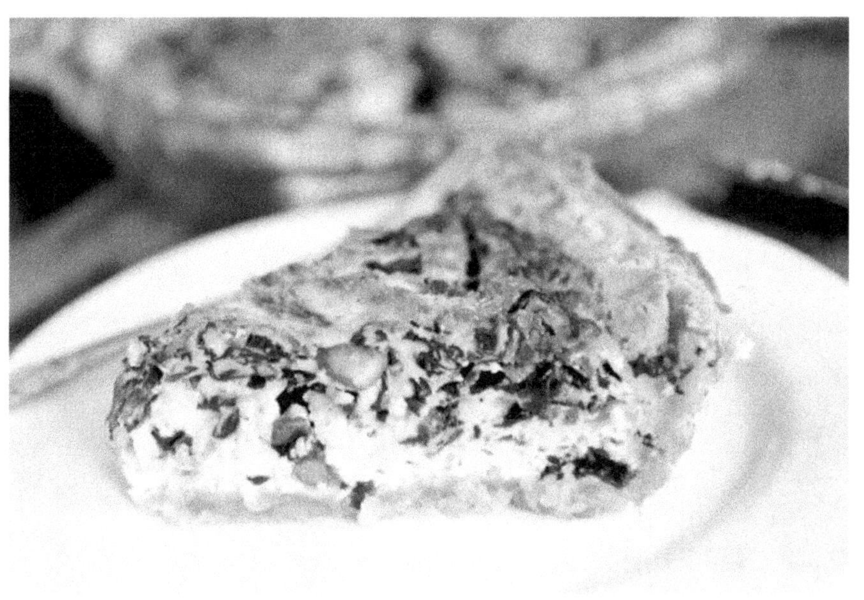

Recipe #18: Cheesy Broccoli Soup

This is a savory recipe that will reheat for a couple days. It will also fill you up every time you have it because the fat between the cream and the cheese goes quite a long way!

What You Need:
- 1 chopped onion
- 4 cloves garlic, minced
- 2c heavy cream
- 4c chicken broth
- 4c water
- 8c broccoli
- 4c cheddar
- 1tsp paprika

How to Prepare:
1) Sauté the onion and garlic first, in a large soup pot.
2) Next, add your liquids. Mix it all together, then add your paprika as well. Season liberally with salt and pepper.
3) Add your broccoli then let it simmer for about half an hour.
4) Next, add your cheese and let it melt. When it's melted, take the soup off the burner, then blend the soup in order to rip the broccoli florets to shreds.
5) Voilà. Enjoy your delicious cheesy broccoli soup!

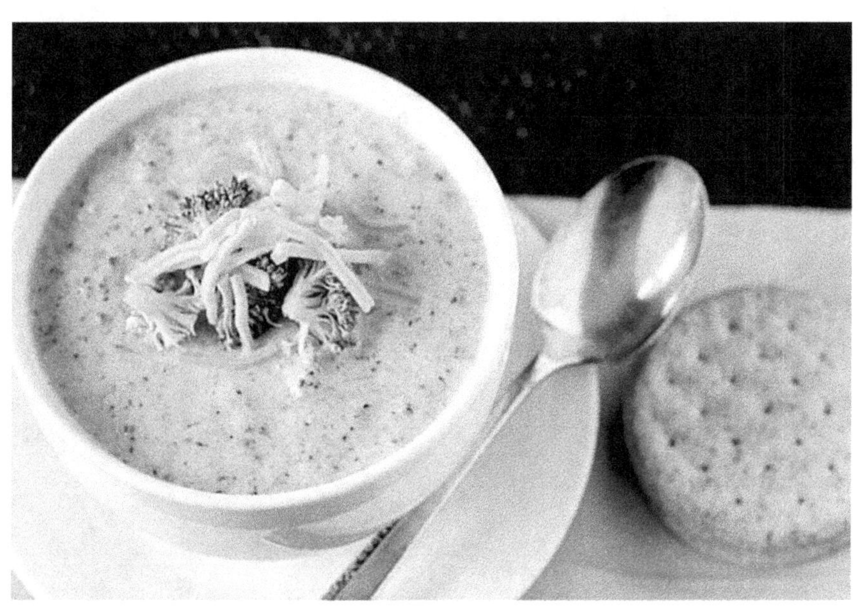

Recipe #19: Burger Bowl

This is a simple and more relaxed recipe, but it still tastes very good and can be reheated over a couple days. Just store the cooked ingredients separately from the fresh ingredients, and you can make it really fast for lunch each day.

What You Need:

- ½lb ground beef
- ½c shredded cheddar
- ½ onion, chopped
- ½ bell pepper, chopped
- mustard
- lettuce
- tomato, diced
- spinach
- 6 strips bacon

How to Prepare:

1) Cook your bacon and then cut it into bits.
2) Brown your ground beef, then throw in your chopped onion and bell pepper with it. Cook it all together. Add salt, pepper, and any other burger seasonings you like.
3) Throw in your cheddar cheese and melt it into your ground beef.
4) Throw your ground beef mixture and your bacon into a bowl with the lettuce, spinach, and tomato. Add in some mustard, too. Of course, you can always add a twist in your burger bowl. Say, fries on top.
5) Enjoy your healthy and super-filling burger bowl!

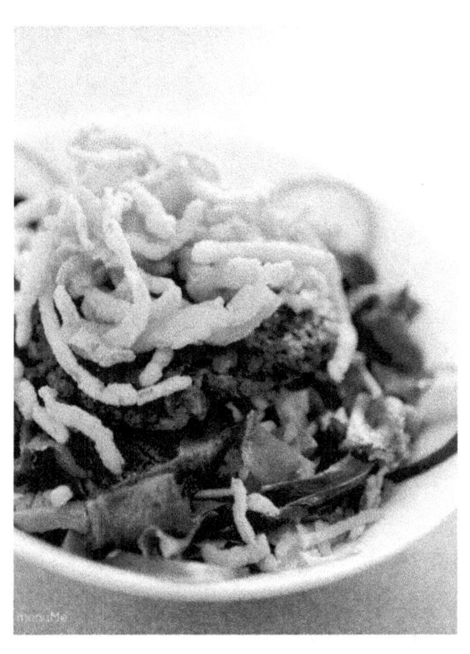

Recipe #20: New York Frittata

This recipe is absolutely scrumptious, and it is also a little bizarre! It builds on a lot of things that we've worked with so far, but it takes them and combines them into a really unique dish. It tastes amazing even if the concept may seem a bit odd, I promise you! And better yet, it's totally keto friendly!

What You Need:

- A dozen eggs
- 8oz bag of spinach
- 6oz of mozzarella
- ¾ cup of ricotta
- ¾ cup of Parmesan
- ¼ cup of olive oil
- 1 clove garlic, finely chopped
- salt and pepper

How to Prepare:

1. Start by warming your oven up to about 375 degrees.
2. Combine everything aside from your Mozzarella. Then pour all of this into a greased baking pan. Top it with your mozzarella. From here, you can add whatever toppings you think might taste good. For example, I like to add onion and sausage. Since it tastes a fair bit like pizza, you can get away with adding stuff like pepperoni as well. Really, do whatever you think would taste good.
3. Pop it into the oven and then let it bake for between 30 and 40 minutes. After it's done baking, you're good to go! Take it out and start enjoying your amazing frittata!

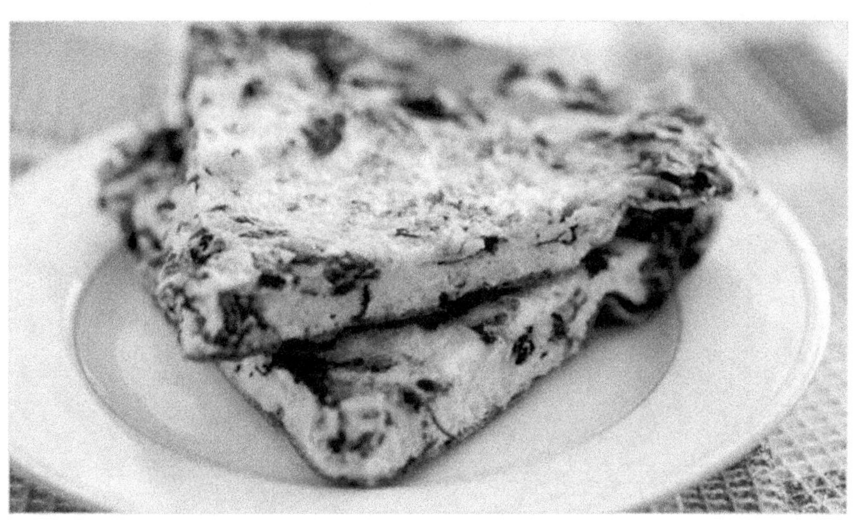

Keto Dinner

Recipe #21: Keto Pizza (Option 1)

When you're on keto, there are two primary ways to make a pizza. The first way is to use a meat crust, and the second way is to use an assortment of different cheeses and ingredients in order to make a ketogenic crust. We'll be covering both since pizza is one of the archetypal American foods. Here's the first!

What You Need:

- 1lb ground beef
- egg
- salt and pepper
- pizza sauce (search store shelves to find the lowest carb one)
- shredded Mozzarella cheese
- Italian seasoning
- pepperoni, sausage, or any other toppings you may want

How to Prepare:

1. Preheat oven to 400 degrees.
2. Get a large pizza pan. In a bowl, combine your ground beef, egg, and salt and pepper. The egg acts as a binding agent to force the pizza to stick a bit more than it normally would.
3. Spread the ground beef mixture all over the bottom of the pan, making it as large of a circle as you possibly can.
4. Throw this in the oven and brown it. This should take about 15 minutes.
5. Take the ground beef "crust" out and top it with your various ingredients. First, your pizza sauce, then your Mozzarella, then your seasoning and any other

toppings. Optionally, drizzle the top with a touch of olive oil for taste.

6. Throw this back in the oven for just long enough for the cheese to melt. Once that's done, your pizza's finished. Slice and enjoy!

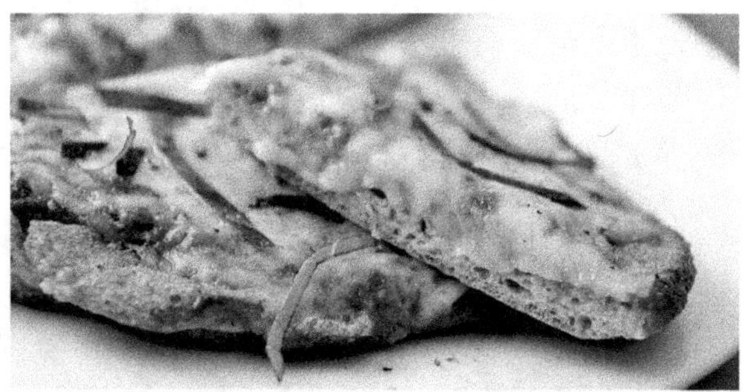

Recipe #22: Keto Pizza (Option 2)

This is the second way to make keto pizza. It's every bit as delicious, and it also offers you a more traditional crust than you would get with the first recipe.

What You Need:

- 8oz mozzarella cheese, shredded (crust)
- 1c almond flour
- ¼c cream cheese
- 1 egg
- 1tbsp Italian seasoning
- Extra mozzarella cheese, about 4oz shredded (pizza)
- ¾c low-carb tomato sauce
- toppings of your choice

How to Prepare:

1) Start by warming up your oven to about 400 degrees.
2) Combine all of your ingredients aside from the extra mozzarella and tomato sauce.
3) Add a touch of salt and pepper, a dash of either (but extra pepper never hurt anybody!)
4) Make it all into a comfortable dough, then lube it up with a little olive oil to make it easier to handle. Then press it into a circle on a baking sheet.
5) Bake for ten minutes, then flip and bake for three minutes more.
6) Take it out and add everything you want, then throw it back in the oven and bake until all of the cheese has melted.
7) Once this is done, your pizza is ready. Cut how you like and enjoy!

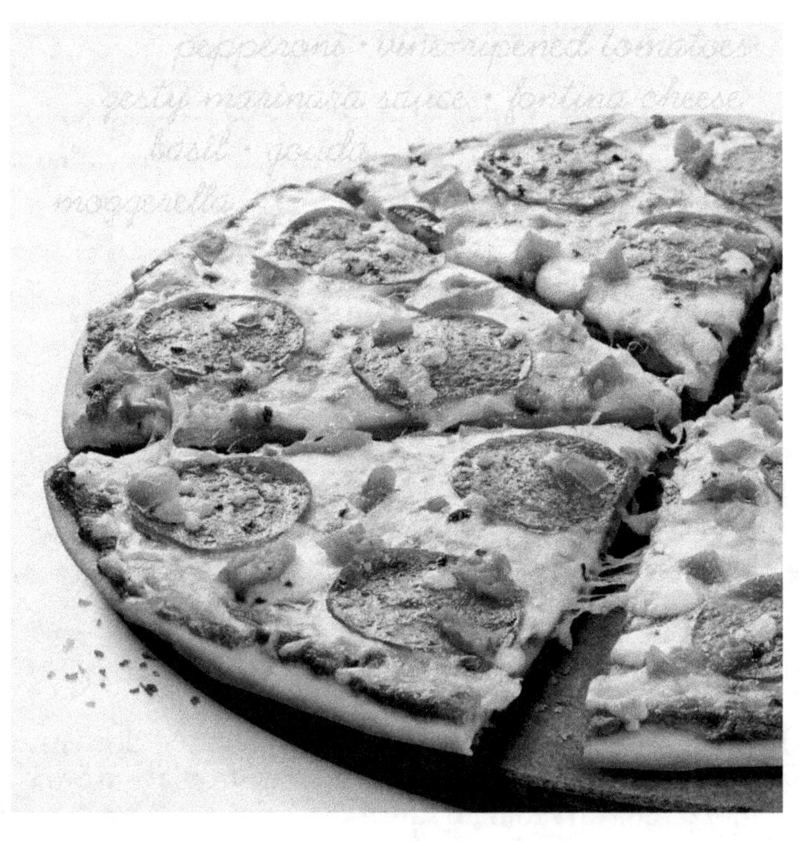
pepperoni · vine-ripened tomatoes
zesty marinara sauce · fontina cheese
basil · gouda
mozzarella

Recipe #23: Mushroom Bun Burger

One of the worst things about keto for me is that I honest to God really like bread. It's probably one of my favorite foods. And there's nothing quite as delicious as a nice toasted bun, covered in butter and fried and then served with a greasy burger between it. It's actually one of my favorite things on this planet.

So it was hard for me to start keto and completely ditch that. However, eventually, I did what I had to. With that said, finding a replacement was incredibly simple and intuitive once I tried to get a little creative with it.

If you want a good and familiar burger with a bun instead of having to resort to the plain ol' burger with a fork and knife, give this recipe a try and see how it works for you.

What You Need:

- 1lb ground beef
- egg
- burger seasoning
- salt and pepper
- Portobello mushrooms
- olive oil
- toppings

1. Combine ground beef, egg, seasoning, and salt and pepper. Split into five ⅕ pound patties and flatten as much as possible since they'll thicken up while cooking.
2. Warm a pan over a burner over medium-high heat. Let heat, then start cooking burgers one or two at a time. Exact timing will vary.
3. Warm another pan and drizzle olive oil on it, coating the pan. Drain excess into the sink.

4. Remove stems from mushrooms as much as possible, then slather outside with olive oil.
5. Toast mushrooms in warmed pan until starting to gain a crispy texture.
6. Place finished burger patty and toppings between two toasted Portobello mushrooms. Enjoy your replacement bun!

This recipe is great because Portobello mushrooms have a neutral taste and don't overpower the burger, but still add a nice bun-like texture and are easy to grip.

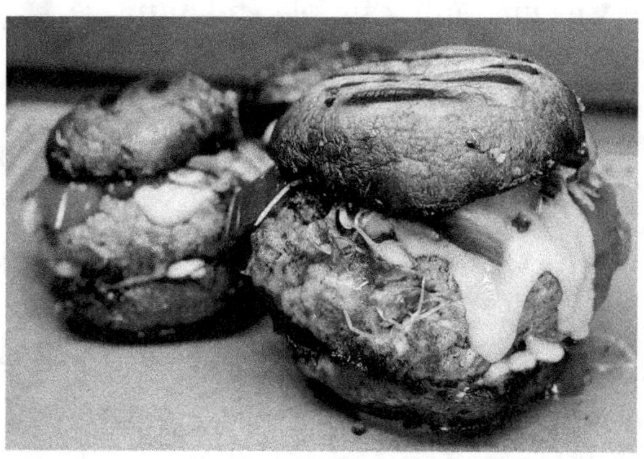

Recipe #24: Keto Red Curry

Who doesn't love Thai food? You may think that you don't get to enjoy your favorite Thai foods on keto since there are so many carby elements. However, here's a wonderful red curry recipe that's totally keto-friendly. Serve it over cauliflower rice for even more authenticity.

What You Need:

- 4 chicken breasts cut into bite-size pieces
- 2 sliced onions
- 2c mung bean sprouts
- 6tbsp Thai red curry paste
- 8 zucchini, spiralized
- 26oz coconut milk
- 4 cloves garlic, minced
- 2c mushrooms, chopped

How to Prepare:

1) Sauté your onion and ginger together, then throw in your chicken. Cook until the chicken is almost cooked.
2) Add in your mushrooms, zucchini, and bean sprouts.
3) Add in your coconut milk and curry paste afterward, then season as you like.
4) Allow everything to simmer. When it boils, you're good to go.
5) Serve fresh and as hot as possible. This makes a *lot* of curry - about 8 servings. Plan accordingly! You can store and reheat curry for a couple days.

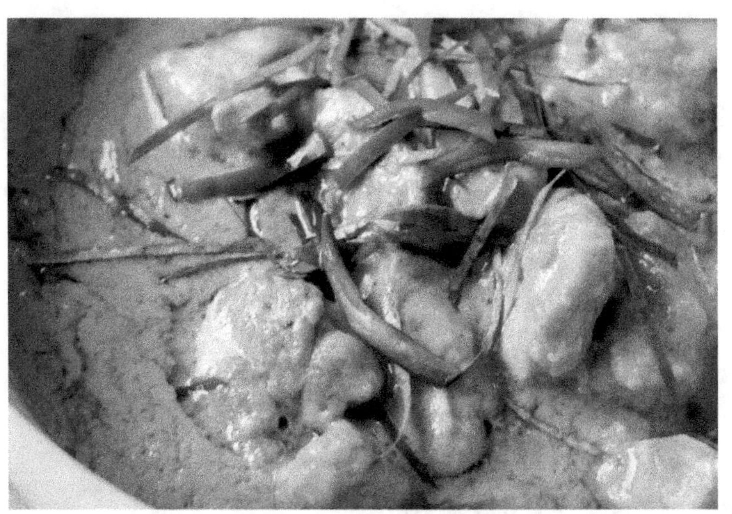

Recipe #25: Keto Mac and Cheese Cauliflower Casserole

If you ever find yourself missing macaroni and cheese, you aren't alone. This cheesy and ubiquitous dish is a hit in American homes nationwide. So what can you do to get your cheesy fix when you find yourself missing macaroni and cheese a lot? Well, this recipe offers you a really easy way to pull it together and make a tasty dish with very little effort!

What You Need:

- Cauliflower, two or three heads worth
- Mild cheddar cheese
- Optional: other cheeses (pecorino, romano, mozzarella, colby, anything you fancy)
- Onion, chopped
- One clove garlic, chopped
- Spinach
- ¾ stick of salted butter
- Salt/pepper

How to Prepare:

1. First thing's first. You need to send your cauliflower and spinach through a food processor together. The cauliflower is what will provide the texture and the substance of the meal. The spinach is just for fiber and nutrition.
2. Preheat oven to 350 degrees.
3. Warm a skillet with olive oil or butter. Sauté your onions and garlic together, then drain excess oil into the sink. Set to the side.
4. Melt butter, however, you'd like. In a large bowl, combine melted butter, onions, garlic, spinach and cauliflower mixture, and a large amount of cheese.

Mix by hand until well blended.

5. Optionally, you can cut bacon and add it to the mix as well. It will cook in the oven, so no worries there. You can also cut chives and/or potatoes and add them in if you want.
6. Throw mixture into greased casserole dish.
7. Layer additional cheeses on top.
8. Put casserole dish into the oven and let cook for 25 to 30 minutes. You'll know it's done when the cheese on the top layer is starting to crisp brown at the corners.
9. Remove from the oven and enjoy your delicious faux mac and cheese!

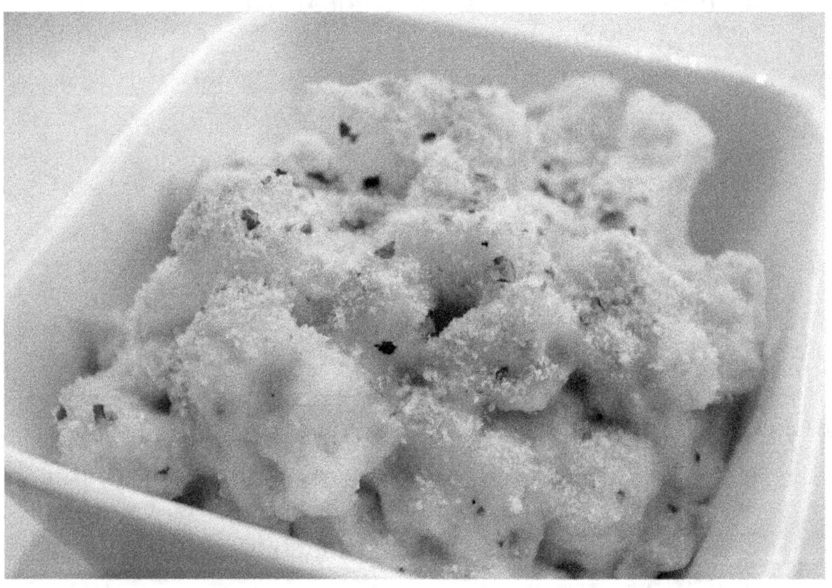

Recipe #26: Eggplant Lasagna

This is yet another recipe intended to help you stave off those darn carb cravings. Keto isn't always easy, but with recipes like this, it can be made easier. This may just be the most delicious lasagna you've ever had, too!

What You Need:

- Big eggplant
- Ricotta cheese
- Parmesan cheese
- Mozzarella cheese
- Italian seasoning
- Sugar-free tomato sauce, with meat, if possible

How to Prepare:

1. The first thing you'll need to do is simply get everything ready. Turn your oven on and have it heating to 400 degrees.
2. Cut the top and bottom off of your eggplant and then slice it lengthwise into thin slices. A large eggplant should yield between nine and twelve slices.
3. Put olive oil on both sides of the eggplant and then bake it for six minutes. Afterward, flip them and bake for 8 minutes. This will roast the eggplant a little.
4. Grab another bowl and put your cheeses in their (aside from mozzarella). Throw Italian seasoning in the mixture as well. Mix this concoction pretty well.
5. Get a pan and then put your sugar-free tomato sauce in it. Not a whole lot, just enough to cover the bottom. Then put half of your eggplant on top of your sauce layer.
6. After this, put on about half of the cheese mix you created, making sure it covers all of the eggplants and

covers evenly. Add a little shredded mozzarella on top of this.

7. Then, you need to throw a bit more tomato sauce to cover, then more of the cheese mixture, then the other half of your eggplant slices on top of these.
8. Repeat the process one more time to finish the dish off: tomato sauce, then cheese mix, then finally a heavy hand of mozzarella to finish it all off.
9. Bake the lasagna for about half an hour, covered with foil. After, take off the foil, then broil it for 5 more minutes. Take it out and let it rest for a half hour before cutting. After that, you're good to go. Enjoy your delicious lasagna!

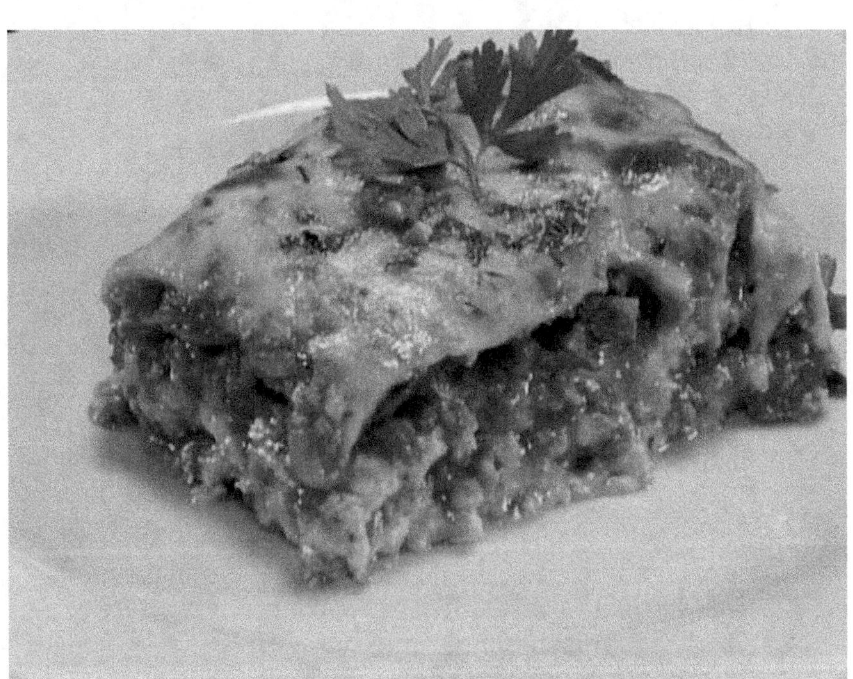

Recipe #27: Chicken Pesto Casserole

This is a really tasty one that you can make. It doesn't take a lot of effort, it will last a couple days, and you can keep enjoying it again and again! It's a great way to set the dinner table, and it tastes incredible.

What You Need:

- Two pounds of chicken thighs, cut into small pieces
- Butter
- 16oz feta cheese
- ¼ cup of olive oil
- 5oz of basil pesto
- 2 cup of heavy cream
- 1 yellow onion, sliced and diced
- salt and pepper
- 2 cloves garlic, minced

How to Prepare:

1) Start by warming your oven to around 400 degrees.
2) In a pan, warm enough butter in which you can cook the chicken pieces. Season them to taste then throw them in and cook until golden, aiming also for a slight crisp to them.
3) Dump your pesto, olive oil, and cream into a blender and then blend it all together.
4) In a casserole dish, put everything together. Then stick it all in the oven and bake it. Half an hour should be more than enough for this dish. You'll know it's done when the dish begins to bubble.

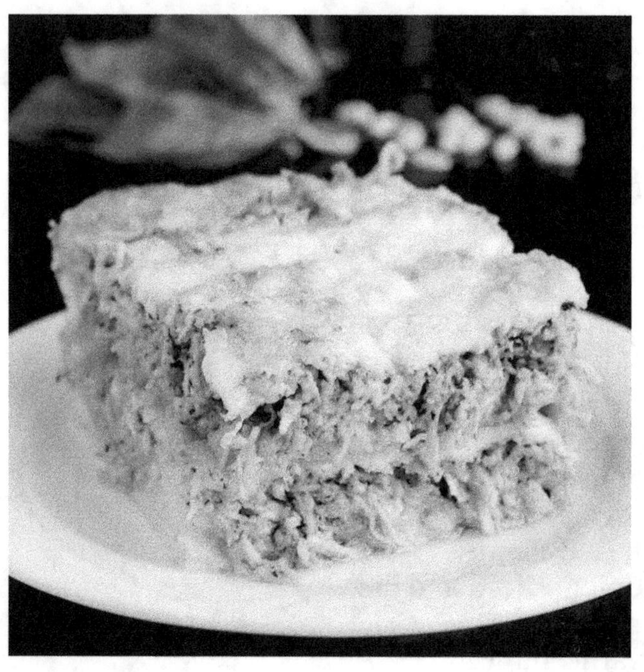

Recipe #28: Keto Chicken Curry

A lot of the recipes in this book have been Italian or Mediterranean inspired. As fun as those are, that palette is very limited! This recipe aims to branch out a bit with some delicious chicken curry. I've made this multiple times, and every time, it's incredibly delicious.

What You Need:

- Unsweetened coconut milk
- Chicken breasts cut into pieces, about two pounds
- Tomato paste, 2tbsp
- 1 yellow onion, sliced (not diced)
- 2 cloves garlic, minced
- Curry powder
- Thumb of ginger, minced
- Bay leaf

How to Prepare:

1) Cut all of your chicken into strips if you haven't already.
2) Get out a large pan that you have a lid to. Warm up some olive oil, about medium to medium-high heat. Throw your onion and garlic in and sauté once it's hot. Once they start to take on a bit of a translucent tone, reduce heat to medium.
3) Add in your ginger and curry powder. It's hard to say how much curry powder because I personally always eyeball this one - I *really* like spicy food! You can always add more if necessary. 3 tablespoons is reasonable to start out with.
4) Sauté everything together, then add in your chicken pieces.
5) Add in your tomato paste afterward, followed by your

unsweetened coconut milk.
6) Mix everything together well. Raise the heat and throw in your bay leaf. Bring the mixture to a boil, then reduce the heat to a simmer and put the lid on.
7) From here, allow it to simmer for about 20 minutes. You want your chicken to be cooked, but not overcooked, so be careful there!
8) When it's done, remove it from heat. You can serve over cauliflower rice - it's absolutely delicious, trust me. From there, just enjoy your lovely Indian food!

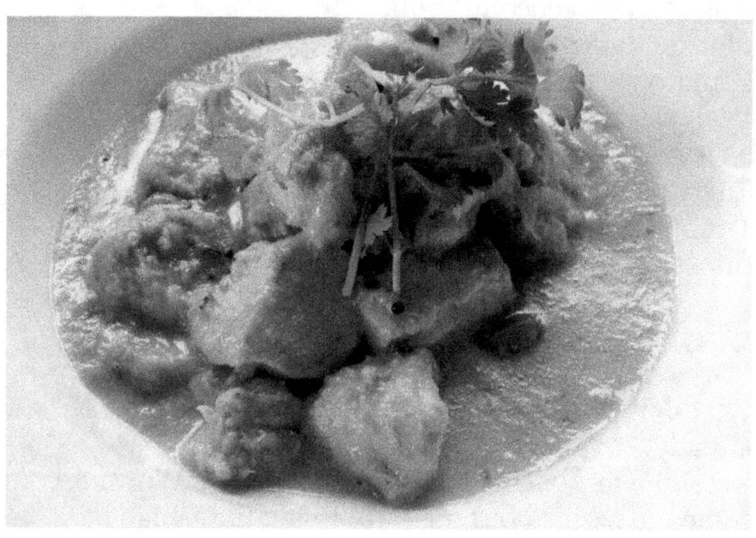

Recipe #29: Baked Salmon

If you want a delicious, succulent, and easy dish, this is the one for you! It's tremendously simple, but it yields a flakey and delicious dinner. Try it for yourself.

What You Need:

- 5 to 6 fillets of salmon
- Olive oil
- Half-stick of butter
- Lemon

How to Prepare:

1. Start by warming your oven up to about 400 degrees.
2. Prep your baking dish by lubing it up with olive oil. Throw your salmon in it with the skin facing the dish. Add a lot of salt and pepper to it.
3. Cut your lemon up into very thin slices and then lay the slices on the salmon. Then slice about half of your butter thinly and lay these on top of the lemon.
4. Bake it for about half an hour. Be careful not to overcook, though - cook it until the fish flakes really easily. When done, remove from the oven.
5. Take what remains of your butter and put it over medium heat. Wait for it to start to boil, then take it off the stove. Add some lemon juice and let it cool. Pour this on top of the salmon and serve immediately. Enjoy your delicious lemony fish!

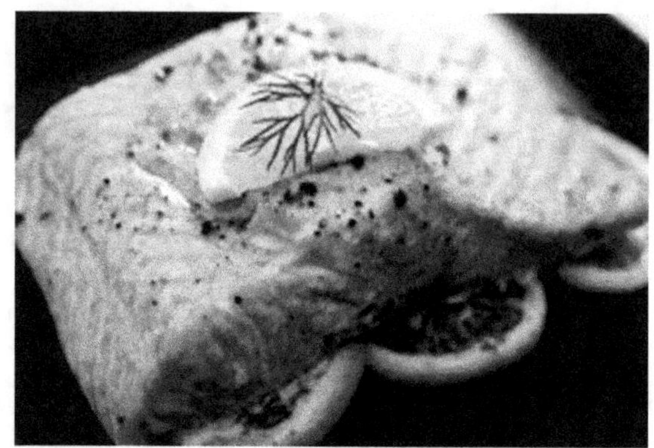

Recipe #30: Keto Asian Skillet

This is a bit of an eclectic dish. However, it's relatively easy to follow and make! What it ends up creating is a bit of a stir-fry. Serve it over a bed of steamed cauliflower rice for maximum appeal and even more fillingness!

What You Need:

- Meat (pork, tofu, and chicken all work fine - easier to cook is better)
- Broccoli
- 1 carrot, sliced
- Thumb of ginger, minced
- Onion, chopped
- Bell pepper, chopped
- 1-2 cloves garlic, minced
- Mushrooms
- Soy sauce

How to Prepare:

1. Start by putting some peanut oil or vegetable oil down in your pan. Sauté your onion, garlic, and ginger in the oil.
2. When the onions are translucent, add in your meat. Raw is fine - it'll be cooking for a while. Also add in your diced carrots, your raw broccoli, your bell pepper, and your mushroom.
3. Optionally, there are other vegetables you can add here. Leek, kale, and chopped celery would all be perfectly fine and add some density to the dish.
4. Throw in soy sauce and a generous amount of black pepper. Stir to incorporate everything.
5. Put a lid on your dish and steam it for a bit. This will trap all of the flavors. Steam until the meat is

completely cooked.

6. Once the meat is cooked, your dish is done. Eat it as is or serve it with steamed cauliflower rice. Yum!

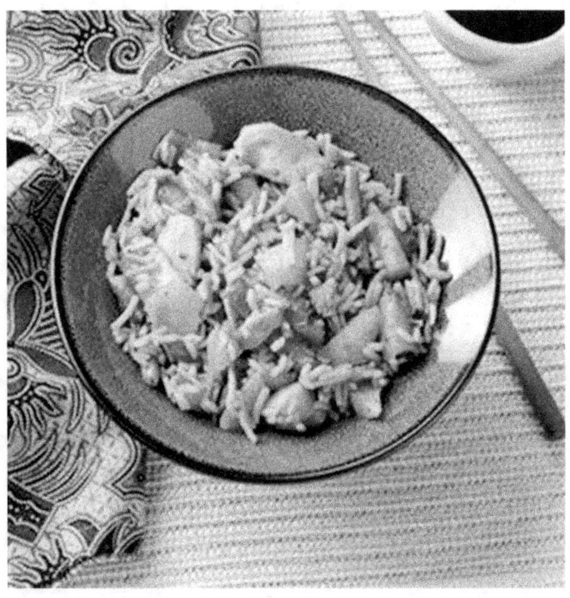

Keto Snacks

Recipe #31: Chocolate Peanut Butter Fat Bombs

One of the most frustrating things about keto is that it's pretty hard to satisfy your sweet tooth, sometimes. These are a lovely snack that you can have which is basically just full of fat. It will tide you over and fill you up really easily.

What You Need:

- 1c coconut oil
- 1c peanut butter
- ½c cocoa
- ½c Splenda
- 1tsp vanilla

How to Prepare:

1) Melt your fats together in a large skillet, then add in your cocoa, vanilla, and Splenda.
2) Pour into molds and freeze until they're set.
3) Enjoy at your own leisure!

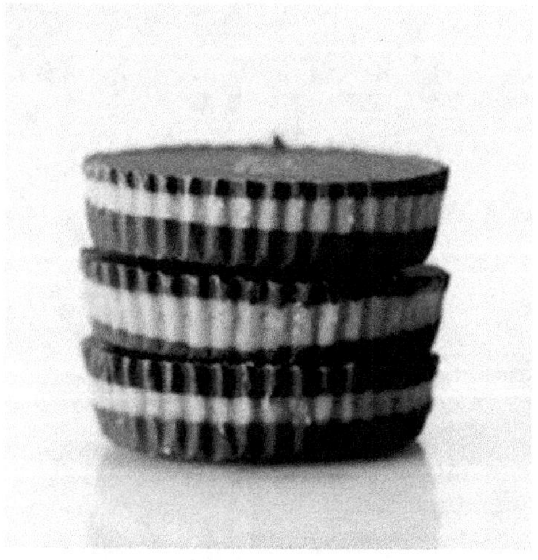

Recipe #32: Cheesy Broccoli

This is a lovable and savory treat that I always like to make after a long day when I'm feeling a bit peckish and in need of a healthy low-carb pick-me-up. It's extremely simple to make!

What You Need:

- 1½ cup broccoli
- ½ cup shredded cheese
- ¼ cup heavy whipping cream
- Salt and pepper
- ¼ stick of butter

How to Prepare:

1. Take your broccoli and place it in a small saucepan. Put a little bit of water in there, enough to steam the broccoli. Steam it with the lid on until the broccoli is tender.
2. Once the broccoli has been steamed, melt your butter into the broccoli.
3. Add your heavy whipping cream, followed by your cheese. Stir and try to get as much cheese as possible to melt.
4. Add salt and pepper, then replace the lid. Let cook for 4 minutes.
5. Remove from heat and serve. What a delicious cheesy treat!

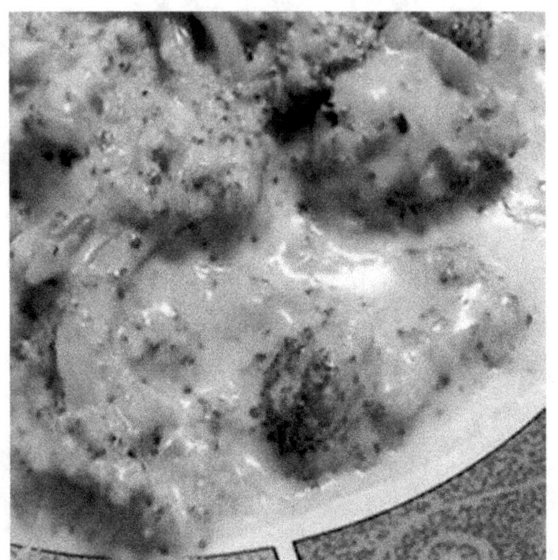

Recipe #33: Kale Chips

You've probably heard one or two people talk about kale chips. Well, they're doing so for a good reason. Kale chips are a delicious food with a lot of potentials. They have all the taste, saltiness, and crunch of potato chips with the added health benefits of kale. There's nothing not to love about them. What's better is that they're perfectly keto friendly; 6 ounces of kale has only 5 grams of net carbs. That's a lot of kale, by the way.

So how do you make this delicious wonderfood? Well, it's easy. All you need is kale, olive oil, and seasoning salt!

What You Need:

- Kale, 12 to 16 ounces
- Olive oil, about ¼ cup
- Two tablespoons of seasoning salt
- Additional seasonings as you like

How to Prepare:

1. Dry out your kale, first and foremost. Rinse it, then throw it in a spinner or wipe all of it vigorously with a paper towel to ensure that you get as much water off of it as is possible.
2. Preheat your oven to about 350 degrees.
3. When your kale is dry, you need to put all of it into a large (gallon size) Ziploc bag. Throw your olive oil and seasoning salt in there, then shake it all up for a while. Make sure everything is coated.
4. Throw it all in the oven for ten or eleven minutes. Watch carefully to ensure that you don't overcook the kale. The center should be green while the outsides are barely browned.

5. When all is said and done, you've got a tasty, crunchy, and super healthy snack. Enjoy!

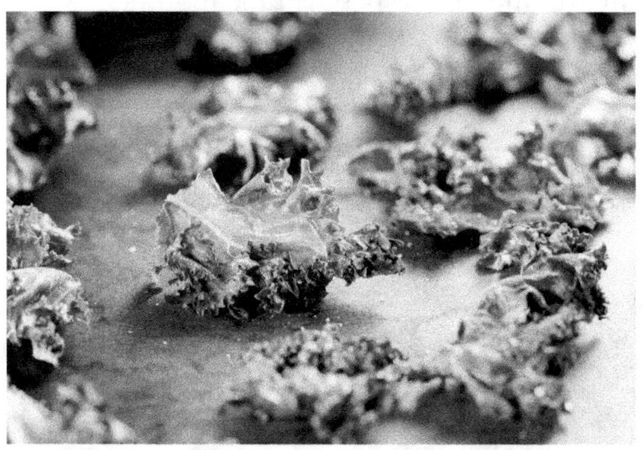

Recipe #34: Keto Onion Dip

Sometimes, you just really crave a good French onion dip, or maybe you're hosting a Super Bowl event and have non-keto family or friends coming over but don't want to make multiple side dishes. Here's a fantastic dip that you and your non-keto family both can use!

What You Need:

- 24oz cauliflower
- 2c broth (any kind, doesn't matter, chicken works best)
- 1 yellow onion, diced
- ½c mayonnaise
- 16oz cream cheese
- 1tsp cumin
- 1tsp garlic powder

How to Prepare:

1) Get your broth nearly boiling then throw in your cauliflower and onion. Reduce it to a simmer and let it ride until they're nice and tender.
2) Add in your spices, and season a bit with salt and pepper, too.
3) Add in your cream cheese and stir until it's completely melted.
4) Add in your mayonnaise lastly, then stir it all together until there are no chunks.
5) Refrigerate for a few hours before having. Serve with things like cheese and celery.

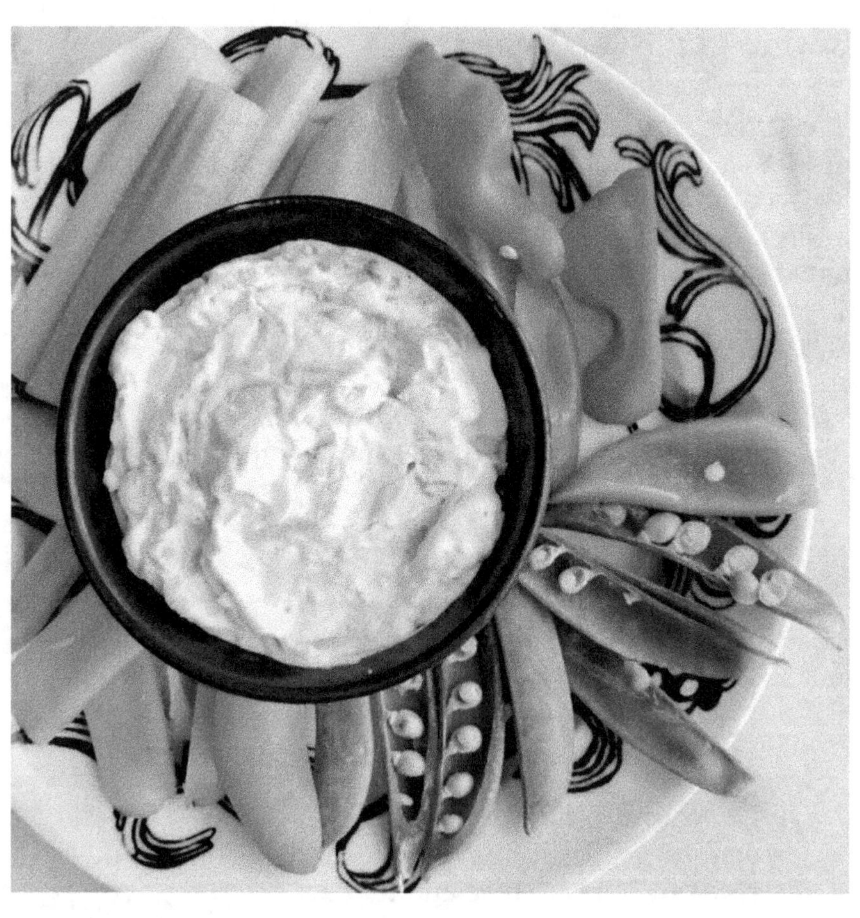

Recipe #35: Keto Burger Bombs

These are bite-sized clumps of flavor that burst into your mouth with delicious grease and cheesiness. You'll absolutely *love* these keto burger bombs. They're extremely easy to make, too! Give them a shot.

What You Need:

- 6 strips bacon
- 6 sausage patties, raw
- 6 cubes cheddar

How to Prepare:

1) Start by warming your oven to 375 degrees.
2) Lay your sausage patties on a greased baking sheet. Season them as you like, then plop your cheddar in there. Wrap the sausage around the cheddar, and you have cheddar balls.
3) Wrap a bacon strip around the ball, then repeat for all of the balls.
4) Put it in the oven for 45 minutes, then remove.
5) When it's all said and done, you've got some delicious meaty balls to eat. Enjoy as you would a burger, with whatever you would put on them!

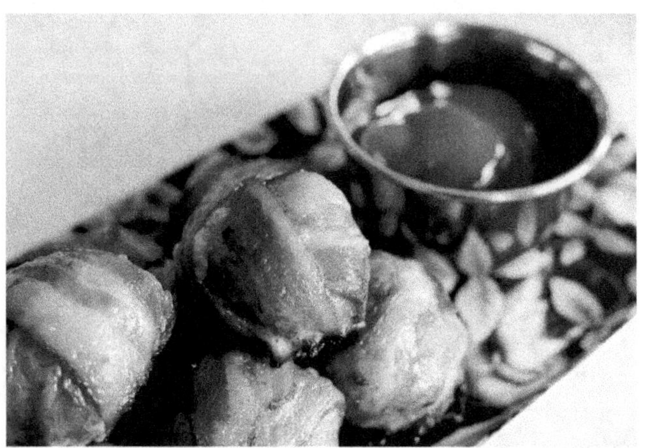

Recipe #36: Mediterranean "Guacamole"

This guacamole is a pleasant blend of familiar Mediterranean tastes alongside the structure of a tasty Latin American dish. Whether you're trying to make a party dish or a dish that will win *yourself* over, this is an excellent snack with hardly any carbs that will keep you coming back for more.

What You Need:

- 2 avocados, diced and mashed
- ½ red onion, diced
- 6oz feta cheese
- 1 clove garlic, minced
- 1c spinach
- Lime juice

How to Prepare:

1) Simply get all of your ingredients together, prepare them, and mix them. You can add many other things for taste, like tomatoes or Greek seasoning. Once everything is mixed, add a heavy amount of salt and pepper to taste as it will bring out the feta and spinach flavors.

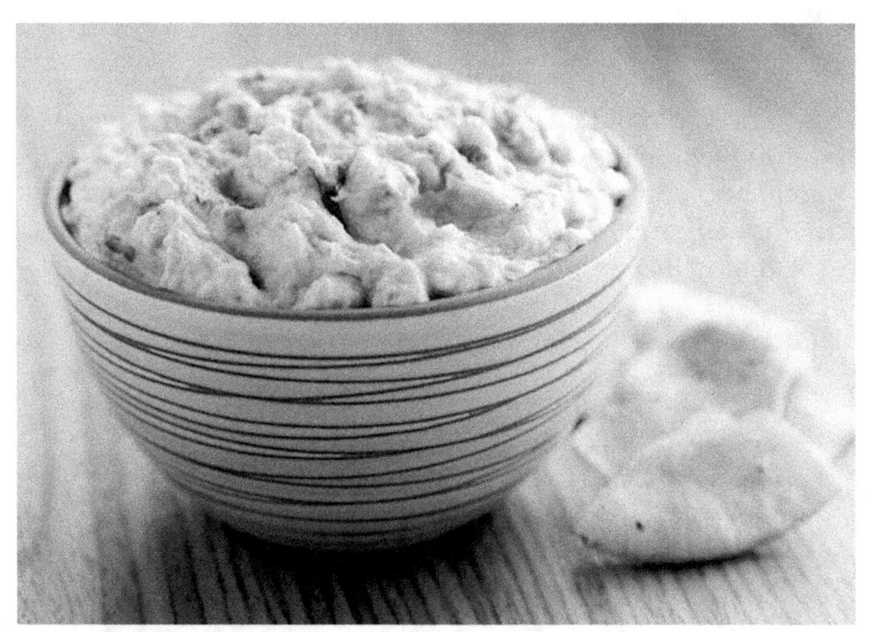

Recipe #37: Neapolitan Fat Bombs

We're all familiar with Neapolitan ice cream, the delicious blend of chocolate, strawberry, and vanilla ice creams into one dish. On keto, sweet flavor blends as such can be a little difficult to find. However, what if I told you there was one sitting right in front of you that was extremely easy to make, albeit a little time-consuming? If you make one batch of these, you'll be set for a while with a fat-heavy snack that will fill you up and fill you with energy, as well.

What You Need:

- 1c butter
- 4 strawberries
- 1/2c artificial sweetener
- 1c coconut oil
- 1c cream cheese
- 2tsp vanilla
- 1/4c cocoa
- 1c cream cheese

How to Prepare:

1) Start by combining all ingredients aside from vanilla, strawberries, and cocoa in a blender, then blending them together.
2) Split this mixture among 3 bowls. In one bowl, add vanilla; in another, add the cocoa; and in the last bowl, add the strawberries.
3) Pour the chocolate layer into molds. This makes a lot of fat bombs, so be prepared for that! Freeze for half hour, leaving other molds out at room temperature.
4) Pour the vanilla layer into molds, next. Freeze for another half hour.
5) Pour the strawberry molds on top of the chocolate and

vanilla layers. Freeze for an additional hour.
6) Once the fat bombs are frozen through, you're all
    done! Pop one out and enjoy!

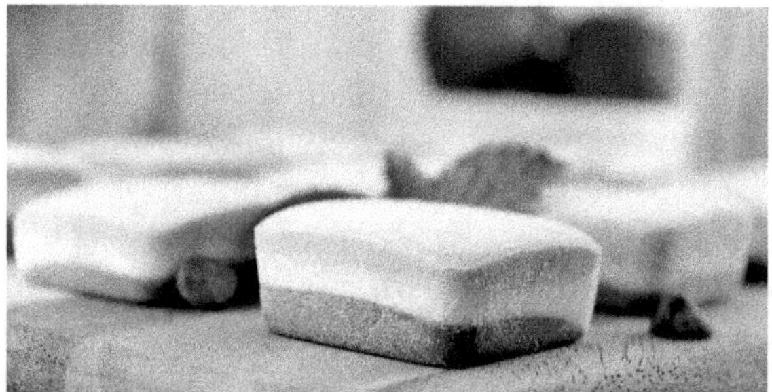

Recipe #38: Keto Deviled Eggs

Boiled eggs are one of the archetypal keto foods because they have a lot of protein and fat, almost no carbs, and they're extremely easy to make, store, and have whenever. Deviled eggs are a delicious way to take boiled eggs and make them even better! Try this recipe.

What You Need:

- A dozen hard-boiled eggs
- 2 strips bacon, cooked and diced finely
- ¼ cup mustard
- 2tbsp green onion
- ⅔ cup mayo
- paprika for serving

How to Prepare:

1) Peel and halve your hard-boiled eggs. Take out the yellow in the center and put them in a bowl.
2) Combine all ingredients with the yolks, also adding a touch of garlic powder, salt, and pepper.
3) Mash together until well-mixed.
4) Put the combination in the bowl into the hole in each of the eggs.
5) Dust with paprika for garnish.
6) Chill and then enjoy! These are a delicious keto-friendly snack that will satisfy your hunger every time.

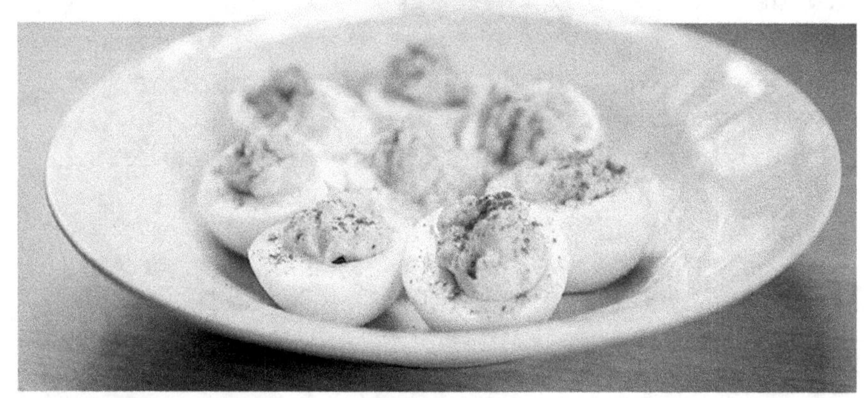

Recipe #39: Bacon-Smoked Gouda Stuffed Mushrooms

Mushrooms pack a lot of utility because they are extremely low-carb and adapt well to the taste of any food. Try this recipe to see just how well they can go with seemingly bizarre dishes.

What You Need:

- 6 Portobello mushrooms
- 6 strips bacon
- 12oz smoked Gouda
- 2tsp garlic powder
- 6 eggs
- heavy cream
- 2 jalapeños, cored, rinsed, and diced

How to Prepare:

1) Start by warming your oven to around 375 degrees.
2) Whip your eggs and your heavy cream together. Eyeball the amount of heavy cream; it should be according to your preference. You're only adding it to thicken the eggs and make them creamier.
3) Prepare your Portobello mushrooms by removing any caps and then clearing as much space inside as you can.
4) Cut your bacon strips, raw, into as small of pieces as you can.
5) Pour a tad bit of your beaten eggs into the bottom of each cup.
6) Combine your jalapeños and bacon bits in a separate bowl. Distribute this mixture among each of the Portobello mushroom caps.
7) Distribute your smoked gouda over the tops of your

mixtures in each cap.
8) Top with a touch of garlic powder, about ⅓ tsp per cap.
9) Finish with salt and pepper.
10) Brush the outside of the mushroom caps with olive oil or butter, then roast it in the oven for about twenty minutes. Broil afterward for 2 minutes to crisp and brown cheese.
11) Take out and enjoy! These will still be good reheated.

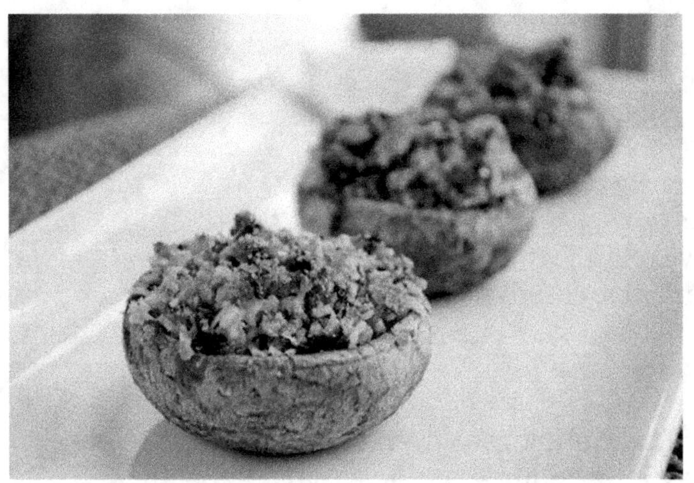

Recipe #40: Keto Nacho Chips

Need a delicious dipping accessory for the French onion dip earlier? Or maybe you have your eyes on a sugar-free salsa that you want to try? These keto nacho chips are the perfect accent to your dips and keto foods - *without* packing on a bunch of carbs!

What You Need:

- 1c almond flour
- ½c flax meal
- ¼c coconut flour
- 3tbsp psyllium husk powder
- 1c water

How to Prepare:

1) Start by warming your oven to roughly 400 degrees Fahrenheit.
2) Combine all ingredients in order to make your dough.
3) Shape the dough into balls then roll. Use a pan lid in order to cut out tortilla shaped circles, then add the perimeter dough back to your initial dough. Keep repeating until you can no longer make tortillas.
4) Cut the tortillas into triangles by cutting 2 diagonals and one horizontal line.
5) Lay the tortilla triangles onto a baking pan, then brush them with butter.
6) Bake until they're crisp, around ten minutes.
7) Once they're crisp, you're done! Take them out and enjoy them with whatever you like. Many salsas are keto!

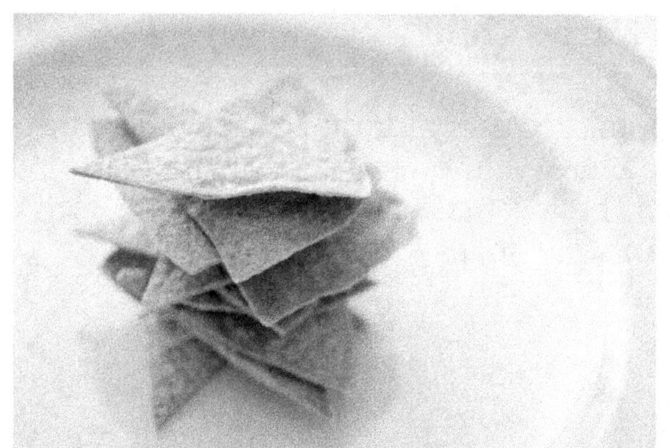

Keto Desserts

Recipe #41: Low Carb Cheesecake

Cheesecake is one of the greatest keto recipes that you can make. Why? Because it's such a fatty and delicious dessert on its own; the only thing that would make normal cheesecake "unketo" is the fact that it has sugar. However, if you replace this sugar with artificial sweetener, suddenly you have a tasty and easy to make dessert that will delight the whole family.

What You Need:

- Pie crust (as mentioned in earlier chapters)
- 2c cream cheese
- 4 eggs
- ¾c Splenda
- 2tbsp vanilla
- 1tbsp lemon juice

  Topping:
- 2c sour cream
- ¼ cup Splenda

How to Prepare:

1) Start by warming the oven to about 325 degrees. Put down your pie crust in your baking tin, springform pan, or whatever you're using.
2) Mix all of your initial ingredients together. In a separate bowl, mix your sour cream and Splenda.
3) Throw the initial mixture into your baking tin and spread it evenly over your crust. Put the cheesecake in the oven for half an hour. Take it out and allow it to cool for another half hour.
4) After it's cool, spread your sour cream topping over the top and then sprinkle pumpkin pie spice, nutmeg, or cinnamon over the top.

5) Let it sit overnight if you can wait, as it will taste better. Then slice into it and enjoy!

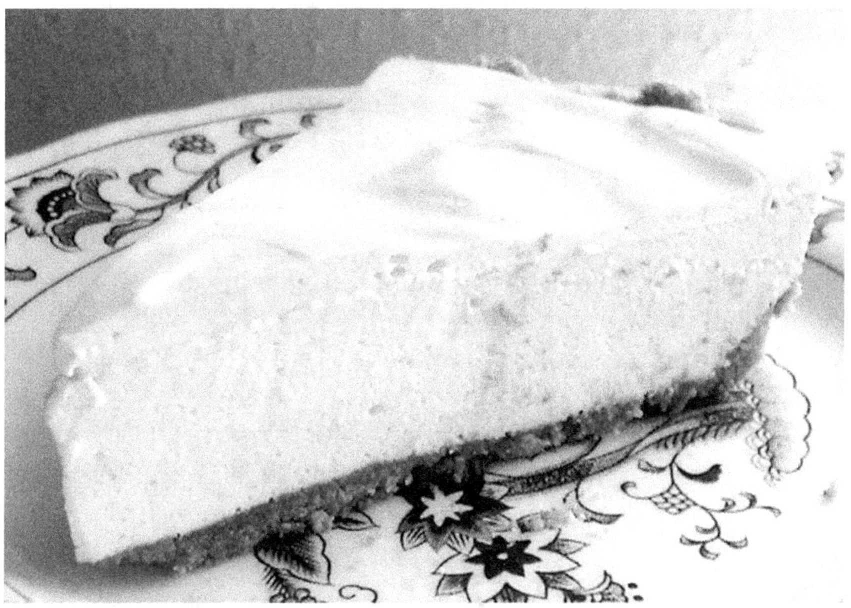

Recipe #42: Coconut Cocoa Cookies

These scrumptious cookies are guaranteed to be an instant hit, even with your non-keto family members. Every time I make these, I get a huge number of compliments on how delicious they are. As a proud keto-er, it makes my heart (and my stomach!) feel very full. If you want to make these amazing cookies for yourself, then here's how.

What You Need:

- 1½ cup almond flour
- ¾ cup baking chocolate pieces (chips or nibs)
- ¾ cup coconut flakes
- 1 cup Splenda
- ¾ cup almond butter

- ½ cup butter
- 3 eggs

How to Prepare:

1) Start by warming your oven to around 350 degrees. In a bowl, combine your dry ingredients, along with a pinch of salt.
2) In a bowl, melt and combine all wet ingredients.
3) Combine all of your wet and dry ingredients.
4) Spoon out cookies onto your baking sheet - this recipe will make about 20.
5) Flatten the cookies then bake them for about twenty minutes. Remove them and let cool.
6) Once the cookies are cooled, enjoy them! These are incredibly tasty cookies that will make your mouth water just by their smell.

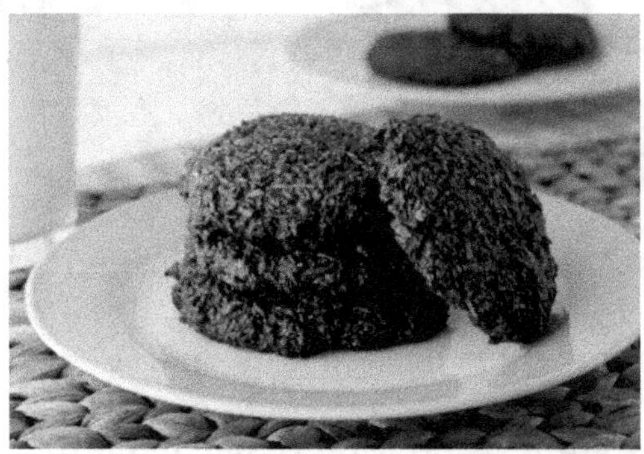

Recipe #43: Delicious Peanut Butter Balls

One of my favorite candies before going on keto was Reese's. While in the last chapter we made fat bombs that somewhat loyally approximated a good peanut butter cup, these go one step further and don't have the "dull" fatty taste that the fat bombs do. Give these a shot! They'll most certainly satisfy your sweet tooth.

What You Need:

- ½c peanut butter
- ¼c cocoa powder
- ¼c Splenda
- 2tbsp almond flour
- 1c coconut shreds

How to Prepare:

1) Mix all things together aside from the coconut shred.
2) Freeze for around two hours.
3) Spoon out the mix, round it into a ball, then coat it with your coconut shreds.
4) Place the balls in the fridge so that they can become firmer.
5) Enjoy the balls when they're finished - they're absolutely delicious! Feel free to accent with a touch of sea salt for some extra charm.

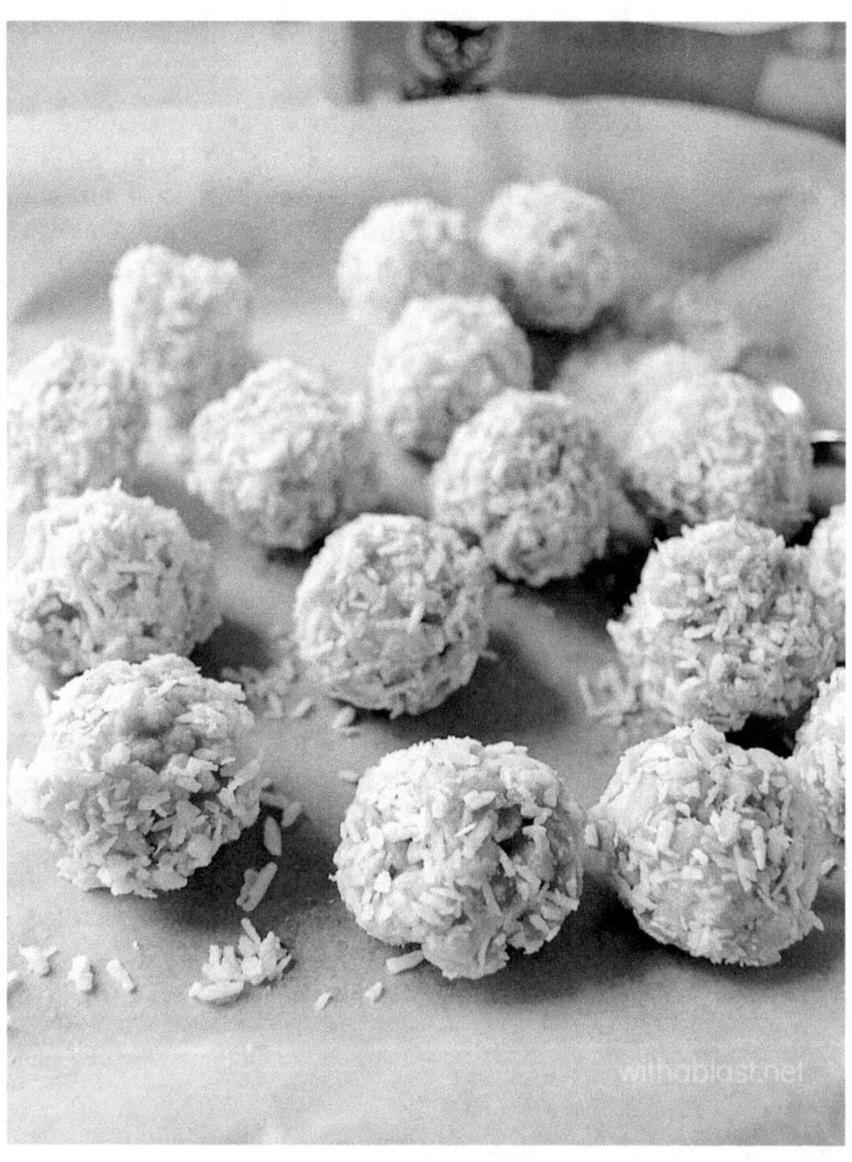

Recipe #44: Keto Chocomocha Mousse

This delicious mousse is a fantastic dessert dish. It's also very tasty and sweet and will satisfy any sweet tooth, no questions asked.

What You Need:

- 2c cream cheese
- 2tbsp instant coffee
- ½c sour cream
- ¼c butter
- ½c cocoa
- 1tbsp vanilla
- ⅔c Splenda
- Cool whip

How to Prepare:

1) Mix all ingredients together aside from cool whip. Then, fold in cool whip. Put it in serving cups and then chill until ready to serve, which should take around three hours.
2) Take it out when set and enjoy!

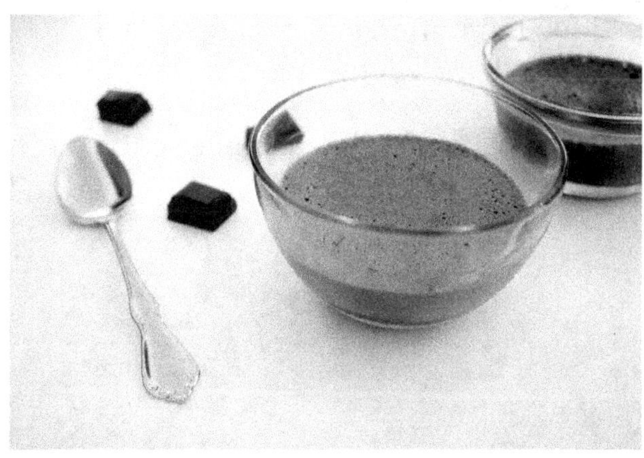

Recipe #45: Keto Pound Cake

Strawberries are keto-friendly. Whipped cream is keto-friendly. Unfortunately, pound cake isn't. Or is it? With this pound cake recipe, you can start to have delicious strawberry shortcake without any of the carby-guilt - or any number of *other* things you may use it for! It even tastes good enough that you could enjoy it all on its own. It makes a *lot*, so be prepared!

What You Need:

- 5c almond flour
- 1c unsalted butter
- 3c Splenda
- 16 eggs
- 1tbsp vanilla
- 2tsp lemon zest
- Salt
- 2c cream cheese
- 1tbsp baking powder

How to Prepare:

1) Start by warming the oven to around 350 degrees.
2) In a big bowl, put your butter, cream cheese, and Splenda. Blend together well, then add in every other ingredient. Blend until smooth.
3) Bake for an hour and a half. When it comes out, you're ready to enjoy this delicious cake!

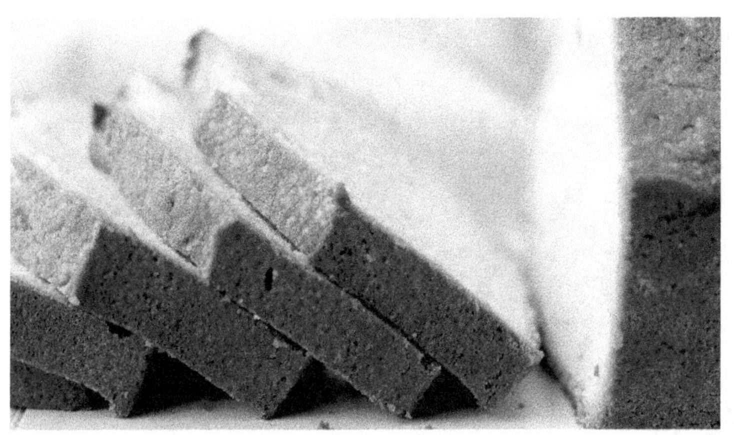

Recipe #46: Lemon Poppyseed Soufflé

This recipe is fantastic because it is a marvelous springy dessert with a lot of pep to it. It's rich and really great on the taste buds as well.

What You Need:

- 2c ricotta
- ½c Splenda
- 4tsp lemon zest
- 4 eggs
- 1tbsp vanilla
- 1tbsp poppy seeds
- 2tbsp lemon juice

How to Prepare:

1) Start by warming your oven to around 375 degrees.
2) Separate your eggs into two different bowls. Beat the egg whites until they start to have a bit of a foam.
3) Add half of the Splenda and then beat the egg whites until stiff peaks form.
4) In the bowl of egg yolks, combine it with ricotta, the remainder of the Splenda, the lemon components, the vanilla, and the poppy seeds.
5) Fold the components together, then put them into a muffin tin.
6) Bake for about 20 minutes.
7) Remove and enjoy!

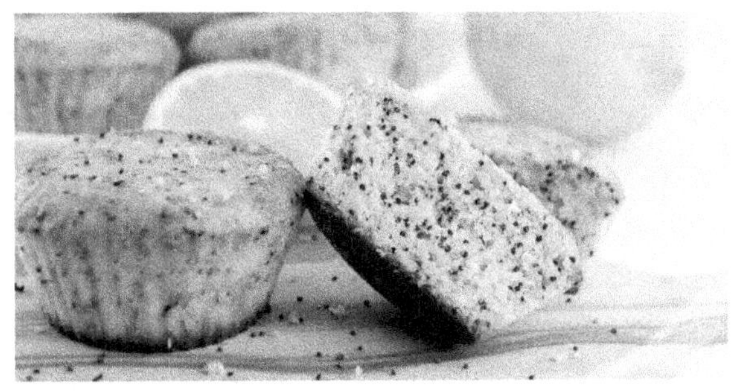

Recipe #47: No-Bake Coconut Almond Bars

This is one of the few recipes in this book that doesn't require you to touch a stove. Just put everything together and then enjoy it!

What You Need:

- 2c almond flour
- 2tsp cinnamon
- ½c coconut shreds
- ½c sugar-free maple syrup
- ½c butter
- 1 cup almonds

How to Prepare:

1) Mix together your butter, almond flour, cinnamon, salt, and syrup.
2) Afterward, add your coconut shreds.
3) Add your almonds, then combine everything.
4) Put them in a dish with parchment paper and then throw it in the fridge. Add cinnamon or coconut shreds on top if you like.
5) Enjoy your food once they're chilled and set!

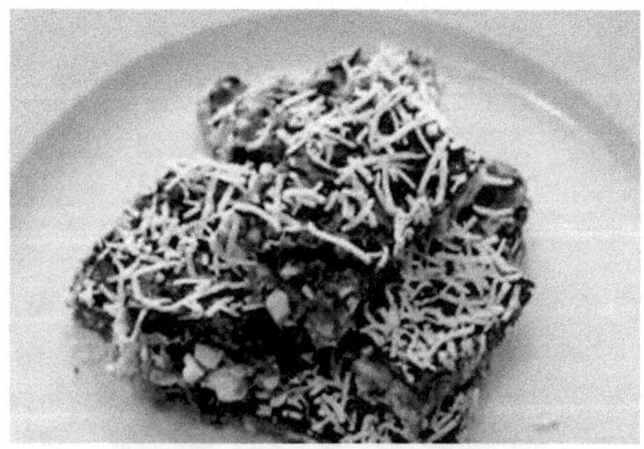

Recipe #48: Hot Chocolate Mug Cake

Occasionally, it gets frustrating not being able to satisfy a chocolate craving because it's such a specific taste. No worries - with this, you can hit that winter sweet spot in a delicious mug cake!

What You Need:

- ½c flax meal
- 2tbsp sugar-free chocolate syrup
- 4tsp cocoa
- 1tsp baking powder
- 4tsp coconut oil
- 2 eggs

How to Prepare:

1) Combine everything in a mug, then throw it in the microwave.
2) Microwave it for about a minute.
3) Enjoy your delicious hot chocolate mug cake!

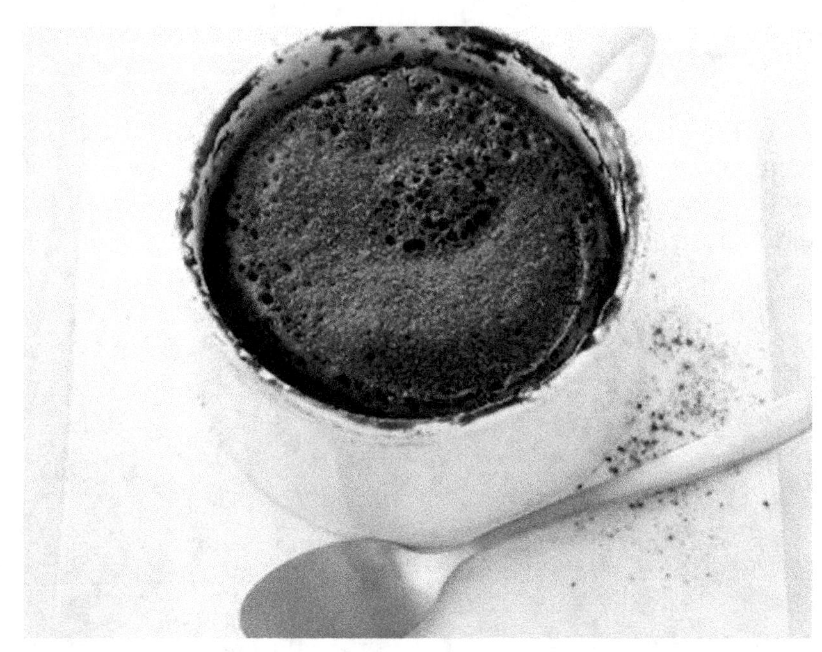

Recipe #49: Peanut Butter Cookies

This is the classic 1-1-1 peanut butter cookies recipe. It's delicious but each cookie packs quite a caloric punch, so be wary of how many you have!

What You Need:

- 1c peanut butter
- 1c Splenda
- 1 egg

How to Prepare:

1) Start by warming the oven to about 350 degrees.
2) Combine all ingredients in a big mixing bowl, then press them on a greased baking sheet.
3) Compress them with the lattice-fork peanut butter design, by just pressing them with a fork in a crisscross.
4) Bake in the oven for 15 to 20 minutes, then take them out and let cool.
5) After cooling, enjoy your delicious and simple peanut butter cookies!

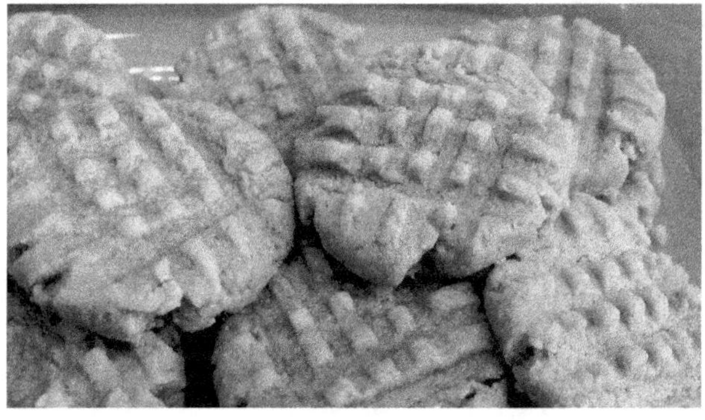

Recipe #50: Pumpkin Pie Pudding

Here comes Thanksgiving. It may be frustrating that you can't eat pumpkin pie with everybody else. However, you can enjoy this, instead! You can maybe even top it with a bit of whipped cream for authenticity.

What You Need:

- ⅔c Splenda
- 3c whipping cream
- 1tsp pumpkin pie spice
- ½c pumpkin puree
- 6 egg yolks (no whites)
- 2tsp vanilla

How to Prepare:

1) Grab a saucepan. Within it, combine your dry ingredients. Then, add your wet ingredients, slowly adding in your whipping cream last, whisking slowly.
2) Heat it slowly until it thickens. It'll take around five minutes. After it has become thick, put it in a bowl and then refrigerate it. Mix it every 15 minutes or so.
3) After setting for a couple hours, you can take it out and chow down on your delicious pumpkin pie pudding.

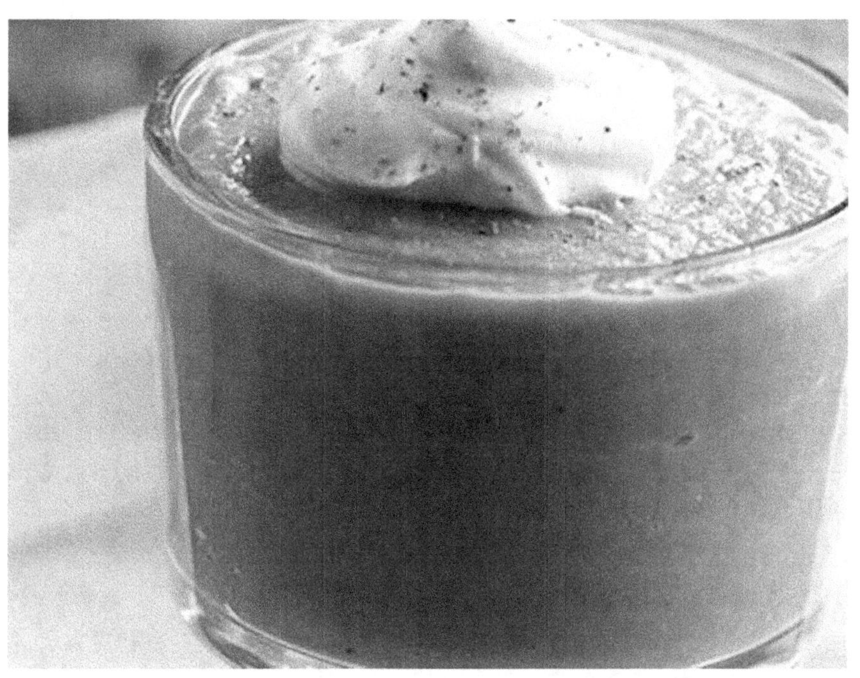

Conclusion

Thanks for making it through to the end of *Ketogenic Diet: The Best Ketogenic Recipes to Lose Weight*, let's hope it was informative and able to provide you with all of the tools you need to achieve your goals whatever it may be.

As you can see, you do not have to be strict on yourself to achieve a slim and healthy body. Ketogenic Diet is not like the other fad diet plans that will force you to digest something that you do not like. The recipes shown in this book prove that you can still lose weight while enjoying the foods that you like.

Of course, losing weight does not happen overnight. And it's not that easy. You have to exert physical effort – and by physical effort, I mean doing physical exercises. You do not have to jump right into extreme workouts. You can start by doing light movements.

The food you take is very important to your overall well-being. When you eat unhealthy foods, your body tends to become unhealthy as well. Not just that, you will also gain weight. So, you have to be very picky of what you eat. The recipes in this book will help you in making great and unique meals throughout the day.

So, the next step is to start making these and speed up your weight loss with incredible food! Pick a recipe you'd like to try, go to the grocery store and buy the ingredients, and then follow the instructions.

Finally, if you found this book useful in any way, a review on Amazon is always appreciated!

www.ingramcontent.com/pod-product-compliance
Lightning Source LLC
Chambersburg PA
CBHW050928260726
48660CB00001B/447

9 781981 696123